With this illuminating volume,
you'll learn to:
- ✧ pace yourself
- ✧ conquer fear
- ✧ overcome force with softness
- ✧ follow your bliss
- ✧ channel your energy
- ✧ free your mind of anger, fear,
       guilt, and hatred
- ✧ safeguard strength
- ✧ gain self-respect
- . . . and much more.

"Drawing from his basis in the martial arts, Joe Cardillo guides the reader through an exciting passageway of new discoveries—ultimately leading to a more refined method of encountering and interacting with life."

—Scott Shaw, author of *Nirvana in a Nutshell* and
The Warrior Is Silent: Martial Arts and the Spiritual Path

"Delivers ancient tools for living well. This book will teach you how to walk in the world like a martial arts master."

—Fred Miller, author of *How to Calm Down*

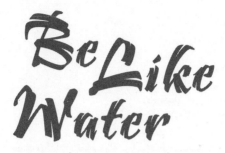

Be Like Water

Practical Wisdom from the Martial Arts

Joseph Cardillo

WARNER BOOKS

NEW YORK   BOSTON

Warner Books
Hachette Book Group USA
1271 Avenue of the Americas
New York, NY 10020

Visit our Web site at www.HachetteBookGroupUSA.com.

Printed in the United States of America

First Edition: September 2003
10 9 8 7 6 5 4

Warner Books and the "W" logo are trademarks of Time Warner Inc. or an affiliated company. Used under license by Hachette Book Group USA, which is not affiliated with Time Warner Inc.

Library of Congress Cataloging-in-Publication Data
Cardillo, Joe.
    Be like water : practical wisdom from the martial arts / Joseph Cardillo.
    p. cm.
    ISBN 0-446-69031-7
    I. Martial arts—Philosophy. 2. Martial arts—Psychological aspects.
    I. Title.

GV1101.C37 2003
796.8'01—dc21

2003041068

Cover design by Brigid Pearson
Cover photo by David Trood Pictures / The Image Bank
Book design and text composition by Ellen Gleeson
Author photo by E. McHenry

For my wife,
Elaine,
and our household of little creatures:
Mignonne, Russé, Sharona, Jolie, Albinoni, Celia,
and Elsa

Acknowledgments

I wish to thank my immediate and extended family for their energies and guidance in helping to bring this project to completion. I further wish to express my gratitude to all my martial arts associates, partners, and colleagues for their support, brotherhood, and sisterhood along this dazzling journey.

Special thanks are extended to Doreen and Barry Bedaw, Alfio and Josephine Cardillo, Alfred and Cathy Cardillo, Maria and Christopher Conover, Molly Chehak, Elaine McHenry, Eleanor McHenry, Matthew Papa, and Michelle Tessler.

And to everyone around the world who believes in the infinite potential of life and spirit.

Contents

Introduction

More than 70 percent of the earth's surface is water. Every living thing is composed of water, and we all need it to survive. Water is a symbol of purity, birth, and rebirth. When you embody the characteristics of this life-giving force, you are going with the flow. You fill every moment with living, you force nothing, you become, you experience, you interrelate. In going with the flow, you become tranquil and peaceful. Ideally, we strive to always and everywhere *be like water*—for water is gentle, and yet it is powerful. It can be still or in motion. It can absorb. It can go over, under, around, and through things. It can dissolve things, float them, or float atop them. It can become hot, cold, heavy, light, invisible, solid, or vapor. It is formless, yet it can adapt to any container. In these pages, you will discover how to become like water. This book is about remaining yourself in an ever-changing world and retaining your sanity in a world full of absurdity. Simply put, it's about going with the flow. Going with the flow is the martial artist's way.

Though martial arts began with the development of language itself and can be traced back more than three thousand years in China, it wasn't until thousands of years later that these combat disciplines fused with philosophy. In A.D. 525, a Buddhist monk from India named Bodhidharma visited the Shaolin Temple of China. What he found was that the monks were deficient both spiritually, in terms of depth and awareness, and physically, in that they could not defend themselves against assailants. Their vulnerability disturbed him greatly.

Consequently, he taught them meditation, breathing, and a host of tenets leading to *a deeper, more enlightened way of life.* He also taught a regimen of exercises taken from the movements of animals, to incorporate into their daily routine. In time, this intense study evolved into an advanced martial arts system known as Kung Fu. Many believe, to this day, that Kung Fu is the core of all martial arts as we presently know them.

Bodhidharma's teachings piloted martial arts from a one-dimensional exploration of combat into a holistic discipline for the strengthening of body, mind, and spirit. Although the element of combat was still significant, the monks who had been trained to avoid conflict were never attackers—rather, they used their skills to help them carry out their work as caretakers and healers.

In the mid-nineteenth century, when the need for fighting skills in the Orient diminished, the focus of martial arts shifted from developing the body for battle to the development of mind and spirit. In fact, it was during this time in history that the word *do* (which means "the way") was added to many martial arts styles. Some examples of this are:

✧ Kendo: way of the sword.
✧ Judo: gentle way.
✧ Tae Kwon Do: way of the hand and foot.
✧ Aikido: harmony spirit way.
✧ Kyudo: way of the bow.
✧ Bushido: way of the warrior.
✧ Karate-do: empty-hand way.

The martial artist's training now emphasized personal and spiritual development: living a better life; becoming a better parent, friend, and human being. Combat maxims were replaced with ideals of self-actualization and welfare, along with axioms such as *Maximum benefit with minimum effort* (or *stressors*).

Martial arts became more about conquering the inner self than about winning a fight. Martial artists were taught loyalty, sincerity, brotherhood, sisterhood, never to retreat, and to look at death unflinchingly—all in the hope of creating a better, freer, longer existence, with the possibility of enlightenment (which involved the transcendence of consciousness beyond their own bodily limitations). Students were taught many ways and means to serve those ends and encouraged to do what worked, not what was dictated by a culture. They were taught *mushin*, which means to empty the mind of guilt, doubt, fear, hatred, and other negative emotions that only get in the way of achievement (or, for the warrior, in the way of winning the fight). They learned ways to increase and develop *chi* (internal life energy) on their path toward self-realization, healing, and power. And they were taught to hand down their wisdom to the next generation.

One thing I have learned in my own quest for a deeper and fuller life is that there are many voices of knowledge: philosophical, theological, scientific, athletic, artistic, and more. No *one* discipline is better than the others. For me, the study of martial arts has been one of the most immediately applicable and successful. In this spirit, I hope to unravel and share some of that knowledge with you. It doesn't matter whether you are a practicing martial artist or not; anyone and everyone can apply the principles in this text.

The process of learning to nurture ourselves with clean, positive energy is a riveting one. You will literally feel your body chemistry cleansing itself. You will think more clearly. You will feel more deeply. You will gain confidence in your ability to take care of yourself. Many amazing things will likely occur. I wish you a warm heart and a joyful soul, strength, and beauty in all the days ahead.

How to Use This Book

Be Like Water is not a how-to guide to performing fighting techniques. It is, rather, a simple study of philosophies within and throughout the martial arts, for the purpose of self-improvement and spiritual development. My aim is embedded in the origins of martial arts thinking, and that is: to put the heart of the martial arts into your own heart so you may return your spirit to its primal state of spontaneity, allowing you to live a fuller and freer life.

Martial artists gain maximum physical, emotional, and spiritual benefit from their chosen art by blending concept with technique—the martial artist without philosophy is nothing more than a street fighter. Thus, each chapter of this text will present a specific martial concept, short narrative illustrations of how the concept can be applied *off the mats,* and daily exercises that I call meditations and resolutions.

The book is designed to be read at your own pace. You can move slowly through its pages, allowing time to absorb the many techniques offered in each chapter. You can also read through quickly and return to those applications most appropriate to current life situations and that you find most immediately useful. Although I have tried to give information that can be readily absorbed and applied, I should emphasize that the pursuit of such processes is a lifelong commitment that will require knowing through personal experiences—each of which sharpens your skills and brings you closer to yourself and the Infinite. The meditations are presented sequentially, but once you've read through the text initially, you can revisit them in any sequence you wish. The resolutions are to help you add richness and positive energy to your life, as well as to contribute direction toward achieving your goals. The ultimate intention of both meditation and resolution is to assist you in discovering ways of adapting martial arts principles to your own life.

You may wish to create your own resolutions, as well. Try writing them out in a journal you keep at your nightstand or one you can bring with you to work or carry in your car. Post them around the house or office where you will see them often. You can also try thinking about them during your meditations or saying them aloud to yourself throughout the day. If you're feeling a little more creative, you can try putting them in an original poem or using them to make a calendar. People who like to draw or take pictures can combine their talents and create several other interesting formats. Don't hesitate to change your resolutions as you begin to grow into the words and live with them a bit. Experiment.

As martial artists all over the world have done, I am passing on in *Be Like Water* what I have learned through my studies and experiences, in the hope that this information will assist you in your quest to live deeper into the beautiful and the positive. Once you have acquired the skills presented in this book, the knowledge will be yours to pass on to others. Each time you do, you will intensify your own understanding of these philosophies and techniques. You will live better, deeper, and more joyfully.

Be Like Water

By adhering to the Tao
Of the past
You will master
The existence
Of the present.

—LAO-TZU

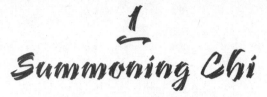

Summoning Chi

Find Your Center

*The entire universe is condensed
in the body.*

—SRI RAMANA MAHARSHI

he Chinese word *chi* (or *ki* in Japanese) refers to our internal life-force energy, as well as to the energy of the Universe, the Infinite, which is present in all things. Everyone is born with a certain amount of chi, and we all have the ability to gather even more. Chi is the core of all existence. It plays into all martial arts concepts and exercises, and forms the ideological foundation of all the ideas in this book.

In everyday life, chi supplies us with the power to break through areas of our lives where we feel stuck, trapped, or limited—either mentally, physically, or spiritually. Chi is the force behind good health, confidence, happiness, strength, power, self-esteem, focus, virility, increased mental effectiveness, and success. It is that thing inside us that cannot be seen; the energy behind all change and self-improvement. It is the power that gives us a sense of safety and fluidity and healing. Ultimately, chi is beyond description, but not beyond feeling or applying.

The major location of chi in the body is within the Lower *Dan Tien,* a space located just a few inches below the navel, and, interestingly, your body's *center point of gravity.* Thus, within each of us is a profoundly nutritious energy, which is the energy of the Universe, the Infinite, and our connection to all things, for everything contains chi.

In martial arts, most of us practitioners will eventually shift our attention from external self-defense movements to softer internal practices of cultivating more chi when we begin to understand that our ability to get things done on the mats *and* in our lives is directly proportionate to our ability to invoke internal strength.

The more we train, the more we heighten our awareness of chi, the more we begin to glimpse its thrilling potential. The power of chi is unlimited. And so, like millions of others, I am enraptured by this phenomenon and have placed it at the center of my training, for martial arts is a way of unlocking the door to chi.

First, you have to find your center. When I began my studies in martial arts, my Karate and Kung Fu teacher introduced our class to the notion of chi early on. I remember he told us to position our hands in front of us as though we were holding a basketball, our right hand on top, left on the bottom, fingers pointed sideways.

"Now," he said, "relax and concentrate on your Lower Dan Tien."

He was teaching us how to *center*. Centering is believed to harmonize the body, mind, and spirit, as well as help in the development of chi.

"Relax completely," he emphasized. "But hold your concentration."

He told us to close our eyes. "Let your weight follow its course downward. Feel the gravity without giving in to it. Relax each joint and muscle. Feel the ground below you. Feel your feet becoming one with it. This is called *rooting*."

Some people like to visualize a cord attached to their spine and rooted into the earth, drawing energy up into their body.

"Let the earth's energy enter you. Breathe deeply through your nose and exhale through your mouth," he explained. "Let the air travel through your entire body— throat, abdomen, limbs."

He asked us to keep our eyes closed and to visualize our breath as pure white, nurturing and healing everything it touched. We began to regulate (measure) our breathing.

"When I clap my hands, inhale," he said. "Slowly."

And with that, he gave us a brisk ten-count. "Now hold your breath." He counted another ten. "Okay, now exhale, slowly." He again gave us a count of ten.

He told us to follow our breath downward and to continue focusing on our Lower Dan Tien. This is the body's hub of energy.

Dating back to the Shaolin monks in A.D. 525, regulated breathing has been taught as a way of increasing concentration during prayer and strength in the fight.

"Our bodies are vessels," my instructor said. "And they can hold only a limited amount of energy, good and bad."

He asked us to continue focusing on our Lower Dan Tien and to visualize our chi as a white light, pulsing vibrantly with each breath.

"Try to extend your chi outward," he said. "Feel it enter your hands. Feel it with your hands."

Regulated breathing, coordinated with the summoning and releasing of chi, helps cleanse the body of bad energy and replenish it with good.

My notion of martial arts up to that point had been focused on external movements and exercises that could be used for building confidence and self-defense and, perhaps, de-stressing. But here was my instructor wanting me to breathe differently, telling me that "internal" concentration would increase not only my overall power of focus, but also my external strength. I was fascinated.

He asked us all to open our eyes. He looked at me. "What did you feel?" he asked.

"I'm not sure." I added, "I felt a slight sense of heat . . . like a warm current."

"That's it," he said.

Many of the other students experienced something similar.

"I want you to remember that feeling. We are going to do a lot with it," he said. "But for now, there is more to learn."

What he was referring to was the assimilation of several other techniques we had yet to be taught that would increase our ability to feel chi and to know when and how to best channel it into our movements.

"For now," he concluded, "just feel it and remember this: Where the mind goes, your chi will go."

Some time after that, I had to stack several cords of firewood in preparation for winter. It was early evening. The golden autumn light had just started to drain from the sky. The air was crisp and cidery and sweetened with the scent of bonfires.

I had set a goal for myself of one cord. It had been a long day, and I would have much rather put the job aside, but there was rain in the forecast. I knew it would be best to stack the wood before the weather made mud of everything.

I remember that with nearly half a cord to go, I decided to humor myself and put one of my martial arts lessons to the test. I relaxed myself, as my instructor had told us. I regulated my breathing. I centered, concentrating on my Lower Dan Tien and envisioning it blazing with energy. I imaged my breath downward, white and healing, flowing through my body.

My labor transformed into a meditation of sorts—not that I thought of it that way. It just happened that way. I soon forgot about being tired and worked spiritedly, continuing the martial arts exercise as I went along. Rather than begrudging my work, I felt comforted by it. When I finished stacking, I felt restored. Instead of feeling beat, I was animated. Not only had I completed the job with much less effort than usual, but what's more, I felt generally happy.

I had learned that positive energy helps us through tasks and creates joy. Better yet, I had experienced it. I was excited. I started thinking of where else I might apply these same skills. I was confident that I would make use of them in many circumstances yet to come.

Since then, whether I am attempting to strengthen my movements on the mats, conduct martial arts or creative writing classes at the college where I teach, or just increase my energy output for walking, jogging, housework, or gardening, I have used this method of cultivating healthy, positive energy on a daily basis.

Our bodies are vessels. They can hold only a limited amount of energy, either good or bad. Find your center. Cleanse your body of bad energy and replenish it with good. Feel restored. Feel animated. Let your daily work energize you rather than deplete your energy. Create joy.

Meditation
Summoning Chi

Who has realized his true self
gains thereby understanding.
Who has gained understanding
finds thereby his true self.

—Tsesze

Standing loosely, relax yourself (remember, your mind must be relaxed for chi to grow). Imagine a small balloon. Now visualize it directly before you, just in front of your Lower Dan Tien—that space a few inches below your navel.

Position your hands so that they are actually holding the visualized balloon. Let yourself feel this.

Then vanish the skin of the balloon, still letting the air inside it (between your hands) maintain its shape. This is what your chi feels like. Hold it, circulating your hands around its perimeter. Try to increase your sensitivity to it. Feel the pressure it makes between your hands.

Now center; concentrate on your Lower Dan Tien. Keep your hands positioned there so that you can better direct your breath. Breathe deeply and smoothly. Regulate your breathing to a brisk ten-count. If a count of ten is too strenuous, try five or less until you can work your way up.

Hold your breath, also for a brisk ten-count, then slowly release it.

Draw your breath down to your Lower Dan Tien and feel the energy gathering there. Feel yourself drawing energy up from the earth. Let that energy also gather in your Lower Dan Tien. Likewise, let the energy of the cosmos enter through your Upper Dan Tien (the chakra point at the top of your head). Let it, too, flow and gather to where you are holding your hands.

Visualize the energy flowing into you and your chi building below your hands. Use deep breathing to direct your chi anywhere you wish it to go within your body. Your hands can also help direct it if necessary. First, flick your fingers, to get your chi circulating. Then touch them to the location you are attempting to invigorate and strengthen, so that you create a target where you can direct your breath. Feel the clean, nutritious, and healing energy.

Speak to your body. Ask it what it needs in terms of physical, emotional, and spiritual nutrients. Imagine your body's answers as planes of color. Your job is to translate what the color means to you in terms of physical, emotional, and spiritual foods.

You can also focus on your inner voice speaking. Listen to your body's needs and use your chi to send it comfort, strength, and healing. Let your inner voice help you discover and select more effective ways of fueling your needs on a daily basis.

Your centered self is who you are at your deepest. Listen to that voice often. Think and act from a place of balance.

Advanced version. Hold your hands in front of you and visualize your chi flowing outward and gathering between your hands. The energy should feel similar to the skinless balloon. Let the energy stream outside your body. Feel its healing warmth on your skin. Enjoy it. Let it comfort and heal you.

More advanced version. Try moving chi without the use of your hands. Where the mind goes, your chi will go. Be creative; find even more ways to use chi to make yourself feel better, as well as enrich your interactions with others.

I encourage you to combine these techniques with movement—anything from walking to housework, office work, and outdoor work. Also, the smoother the movement, the more fluidly chi will travel through your body. Allow your cultivation of chi to put a luxuriant sense of well-being and strength into your daily routines. Feel the harmony.

Remember, there is only so much energy you can hold. Negative energy will empower your opponent. Vanish it. Positive energy nurtures us, heals us. Use it to help create the life you want. Let it empower you.

Resolutions
Summoning Chi

✧ Today, I will center myself and act from a place of balance.

✧ Today, I will open myself to the goodness of the Universe. I will remain aware that its energy is my energy and mine, its. I will be present to our moving and flowing together.

✧ Today, I will stay centered even in tense situations and watch as my stressors vaporize. I will enjoy the abundance of confidence I gain in myself.

✧ Today, I will look for opportunities to remember that with every breath, I take into my blood the power of the Universe—that with every breath, I must also give myself back.

✧ Today, I will give thanks to the Infinite for sharing with me the power to heal.

2
Emptying Your Mind
Avoid Assumptions

Serenity is the master of restlessness.
—LAO-TZU

ushin, or empty mind, is a calming technique practiced by most martial artists. The point is to free our mind of all assumptions and negative emotions such as anger, guilt, doubt, fear, and hatred. Whether on the mats or in everyday situations, a clear and still mind will react more fluidly and efficiently. We are less apt to chase decoys or get bogged down by actions extraneous to our goals.

Martial artists try to avoid assumptions and negative feelings because they are an all-around losing situation. This kind of mental poison slows you down and even telegraphs your reactions, making you less effective. Negativity makes you rigid, and when you lose flexibility, opponents can easily target techniques around you as simply as water can circle stone.

You want your body and mind to move as smoothly and naturally as possible. Imagine your consciousness as a cork afloat in a stream, reacting spontaneously and harmoniously to any movement around it—alert and light and unfettered.

An old adage says, *If you're looking for something, you will never find it.* The rule in sparring is: *Don't assume you know what's going to happen before it happens.* For me, it seemed that whenever I presupposed that anything on the mats would inevitably lead to a certain end, things hardly ever worked out the way I imagined. I'd throw a kick intended to put an opponent in a blocking situation, for instance, and instead he or she would step back or to the side and return with a flurry of kicks and punches I wasn't ready to stop. I was already in a vulnerable position because of the kick I'd thrown. All I had done was make things worse.

It seemed that whenever I thought I knew what I was doing, even when I did things by the book, I'd wind up getting tagged. Of course, this would only frustrate me, as it would most inexperienced martial artists.

Once, after an aggressive sparring match with another student, my instructor took me aside. "I want you to see something," he said.

We began a light spar. His movements were soft and easy. His eyes were wide and deep like a cat's; they seemed like mirrors—focused entirely on me, alert and yet paradoxically unthinking. This is what many refer to as the martial arts stare. I had the sensation that my teacher knew what I was going to do before I even did it. I could literally feel his strength, and he was *doing* nothing.

"That's the kind of intensity you want," he said.

I knew what he was referring to. When I had been sparring earlier, the kind of intensity I'd shown was the same kind of grunting, growling aggression you'd use to chop wood. That kind of energy is complete intention.

In sparring, you learn that your job is to remain deeply *attentive*, in what could be perceived as a state of active (alert) nonaction. You make no assumptions, regarding your own actions or your opponent's. You have to empty your mind and take each movement as it comes. You open the perimeters of your vision, absorb as much as possible, and when the time is right, you shift—smoothly and fluidly—and deliver your shot.

Mushin keeps us agile—helps us fit in when we want and where we need. A sticky mind is not free to concentrate. A sticky mind is the result of assumptions and prejudgments. It creates confusion where we need clarity. Mushin, on the other hand, teaches us to accept thought without adhesion, like a lake allows images to float over its surface. As a result, we can move and think more freely.

In terms of life skills, mushin is a technique I practice daily. Why? Because it is too easy to start chasing bad thoughts, emotions, anticipations, and so forth, and begin clinging to them. What's more, it's dangerous and often destructive or counterproductive to make assumptions.

Some time ago, I wanted to refinance my mortgage. When I phoned the bank manager, she sounded as though she was stuck in the proverbial bad day. She had absolutely no qualms about dumping her frustrations into our conversation, and, though I didn't react, her attitude troubled me. Later, I reasoned that things like this happen every now and then, especially to people who work with the public all day. But I still couldn't let go of the uneasiness that had been building in me all day over the call, and specifically over the manager's tone.

When my father asked me about the mortgage, I told him the rates sounded good and that I was pursuing it, but that the manager was a rude person. When I heard myself saying that, I knew my frustration was slowly brewing itself into a conflict. I flashed forward for a moment and could see myself returning her rough tone with an edge of my own. I could also see how that would lead nowhere.

When the bank manager and I eventually met, I calmed myself, emptying my mind of any emotional residue from our previous conversation. I chose to void any assumptions I'd made about her. I told myself that this should be an occasion for celebration—after all, the bank was about to save me thousands of dollars with the new mortgage. I met her with lightness and warmth, and she responded in kind. This time, I found her to be a delightfully pleasant woman with a deep smile and a good sense of humor. She was quite professional and attentive. There *are* times when a push can be a functional response to a shove, but this was not one of them.

I had learned many lessons that day—not only that I could apply mushin to life, but also that anger pitted against anger will only yield more antagonism. Furthermore, the assuming mind, allowed to run loose, will contaminate relationships and limit successes.

Eliminating negative emotions and assumptions is difficult for everyone, but there are great benefits to be achieved as soon as we begin trying. The trick is to flow with the situation, not control it. Give yourself permission to let go of negativity. Don't trust it. It works against you.

Practice mushin. Empty your mind of emotional residue and unyielding reactions. Anger is your enemy. Avoid assumptions about yourself or others. Don't assume you know what's going to happen before it does. Be alert and widen your vision. Practice active non-action. Generate positive energy. Trust yourself.

Meditation
Emptying Your Mind

Do not run,
let go.
Give up thinking
as though
Not giving up.

—Bruce Lee

Close your eyes and visualize someone you feel anger or resentment toward. Let the feelings rise so you can clearly identify them. Next, visualize yourself writing (or actually do this) that person's name on a piece of clean paper. Write slowly. Now, in your slowest and best writing, write down in full sentences what the person has done and how it has made you feel. It's important to write thoughtfully and neatly. If you are visualizing this, watch as the ink feeds itself onto the paper for each letter of each word. Then affirm to yourself that you are getting rid of these feelings because they are only holding you back and restricting your power and appreciation of life. Tell yourself that these emotions will no longer have any power in your life.

The next step should be done outside your dwelling. Tear the paper into little pieces, place them in a pan, and light the contents. Watch them burn, relighting if necessary, until there is nothing left but ashes.

If you are visualizing this process, be sure to take your time, watching as the flames vaporize each tiny bit of paper, as each letter of each word disappears.

Now blow the ashes into the wind.

Alternate version. Rather than burn your notations on the toxic incident and your feelings toward it, fold the paper into a tiny bundle and carry it in your pocket for a day, or tape it to a mirror. Let yourself realize the toll such contamination takes on you per diem—the space it requires, mentally and physically, that you could be using for other things. When you finally burn it, you will take even more pleasure in getting rid of it.

Resolutions
Emptying Your Mind

✧ Today, I will strive for a state of empty mind and generate more space for goodness to come to me.

✧ Today, I will surrender my need to make assumptions.

✧ Today, I will relinquish my need to prejudge.

✧ Today, I will empty my mind of doubt.

✧ Today, I will empty my mind of anger.

✧ Today, I will empty my mind of hate.

✧ Today, I will empty my mind of fear.

✧ Today, I will empty my mind of guilt.

✧ Today, I will empty my mind of shame.

✧ Today, I will surrender the need to control.

✧ Today, I will meet force with softness.

✧ Today, I will choose to redirect toxic energies that are wielded toward me.

✧ Today, I will surrender my need to predict conclusions.

✧ Today, as I open to the utmost emptiness, I will remain safe and whole, and I will be thankful.

✧ Today, I will surrender myself to the Infinite.

3

Being the Flame; Being the Hand

Observe and Listen to Others

All things are our relatives.

—BLACK ELK (1865–1950)
HOLY MAN OF THE
OGLALA SIOUX

Good martial artists don't rely on prescribed moves. These only get in the way of seeing what's actually happening at the moment.

"Try imagining a lighted candle," my teacher once advised me. "Imagine your hand circling the flame, drawing it in or moving toward it without burning yourself. That's how you want to move, naturally and spontaneously. You can be the flame or the hand."

The first time I tried this, I turned off all the lights and lit a candle. The flame was tall and moved in long, smooth lines toward my hand when I began circling it. As I quickened the pace, it followed, leaning in close to my palm, mirroring my movement. If I closed in, it flowed toward me, keeping me in a steady orbit around it. I could literally feel the track I had to maintain if we were going to continue moving together, and if I broke out of this path I would either get burned or lose the adhesion, the contact.

I got burned several times. I had to learn how to move by watching alertly, with a clear mind, and by reacting only to what the flame was doing, not what I presumed it would do. Finding the right path or movement came through *constant observation.* For as long as I stayed in harmony with the movement, I was able to maintain a sense of safety.

I couldn't just observe; I also had to listen to the flame's message. Whether or not I initiated the movement, once I closed the distance between myself and the flame, my hand had to fall into a certain orbit to avoid getting burned. Likewise, the flame gave up its original position and entered into movement with the hand and thus could avoid being snuffed out. It was in this *third* or *mutual movement*—the harmonized or shared orbit—that each was safe. Once in this space, there could be no *my-way-is-the-only-way* attitude because *the way* was constantly changing from moment to moment. Neither hand nor flame was in charge. That attitude had been given up as soon as the movement had begun.

Strategically observing and listening to others creates

an overall sense of personal well-being in our relationships, whether we are on the mats or in the spaces of our daily routines.

The concept of hand–flame has many applications in our lives. Just recently, a freshman writing student of mine had been sitting in class for the first week of the semester with the wrong outline. He had received an outline for an entirely different course. Unfortunately, I was unaware of his situation until I received an email from one of the college administrators. I was puzzled as to how the student had received the wrong paperwork and had worked himself into a panic.

My colleagues advised me to simply give the student the correct outline and drop the issue. And while it might have been more convenient to let things slide, my instincts told me otherwise. The student and I needed to establish an open line of communication. After all, for whatever reason, he had felt more comfortable discussing his problem with someone else rather than me—behavior that could create future problems.

Although my colleagues had expressed concern that the situation was somewhat delicate because the student was already animated, I gently went ahead. I focused on defusing any confrontation.

I gathered my energy and made sure I was cooled off. I did my best to clear my mind of any preconceived judgments, remaining open for any opportunity to enter into what would be our third movement. I softened my demeanor and initiated action by mentioning I'd heard about the confusion in outlines, adding quite naturally that I would set him up with the correct paperwork. I tried to remain as alert and unassuming as possible.

Interestingly, his mood lightened ever so slightly when I mentioned getting him what he wanted, which was the right outline. That was my opening. I'd started a new movement, and he'd gravitated into it. I asked him how he had received the incorrect materials, and he told me that he had missed the first class—perhaps that had had something to do with it. Now we were in a common orbit.

I lightly responded, "Well, yes," but added that he wasn't entirely responsible in that I had inadvertently handed him the wrong paperwork at a busy moment. We were moving in harmony, and I could *feel* the positive direction our conversation was now headed. We had discovered the third movement. It offered a sense of well-being—advantageous for both of us.

Don't stop. Keep observing and listening even though things take a turn to your advantage. In this situation, my student really loosened up and started telling me about how he'd panicked and gone to an administrator, fearing he'd been scheduled into the wrong class. He was expending his anxieties along the way. Then I saw what he really needed:

"It must have been rough," I said. "I mean, to have to sit there for that long—that confused." I had a hunch that this was really causing his anxiety, and I wanted to let him know that I understood. That's what harmony does. Besides smoothening your movements, it helps create compassion and peace.

He looked at me, visibly relieved, and quietly nodded. He went on to tell me about all the assignments—the wrong assignments—he'd been doing in advance. He assured me that he'd be all right from that point on, and we parted, having both gotten what we needed. The lines of communication had opened, and they remained that way.

It's not always easy to initiate action that helps transport and sustain two or more misaligned people onto a mutual path. With practice and heightened states of attention, however, these paths will often reveal themselves. As we strive to empathize and become more compassionate with those around us, they will begin to open up to us more freely and generously. We will notice our relationships getting more comfortable and peaceful, rather than distancing and creating anxiety.

Yet desire alone cannot change the course of a relationship. We must remember to observe and listen to others. This allows truth to surface naturally and without conflict. For like the flame and the hand, we empower each other when our actions and reactions evolve from harmony rather than discord. The attitude with which we approach each other will be nurturing, compassionate, and respectful—which will allow us to see more clearly how to create responses that will gather more goodness and love into our lives. We will become light and less conflicted. We will see more goodness in others and they in us. Our actions will work toward lightening their load and theirs toward lightening ours.

Don't rely on prescribed reactions. Have patience. There is no need for forcing solutions. There is no need to dominate. Gentleness will safeguard strength. Observe and listen to others. In harmony, leading and being led become the same movement. Direction is spontaneous. Be the flame. Be the hand. Harmonize. What you need will come to you. Respect others. Enjoy your gained respect. Feel safe. Feel good.

Meditation
Being the Flame; Being the Hand

*Through harmony
all things are influenced.*

—Confucius

The following meditation works wonderfully in a dimly lighted room. Start by lighting a candle, preferably one with a wick that will allow for a long flame. Next, hold your hand so that your palm is facing the flame and close enough so that you can feel its warmth. Then, slowly, begin to move your hand in a circle around the flame. Stay close enough to feel its heat.

Avoid direct contact with the flame itself. Your objective is to set the flame in motion, allowing it to not only follow your hand, but also to lean in and out of your movement—in essence creating the path of movement *with* you.

Try to feel (rather than think) the path it reveals to you as you attempt to sustain contact. Remain as attentive as possible. Let yourself feel the harmony of the movement as it evolves from moment to moment. Let yourself trust in the safety and harmony of your ability to feel.

Advanced version: Here is a visualization you can try. Call to mind someone in your life who has become a source of tension. Consider a specific source of conflict you are experiencing with that person. Visualize yourself in a setting in which you commonly encounter each other. Recall the movement of your hand around the flame. Recall the movement of the flame as it leaned into the energies of your hand. Imagine yourself in a relaxed yet alert state of empty mind. This is important because in this form, your thoughts become infinitely more capable. Observe and listen to yourself interacting with the other person. Observe and listen to the other person interacting with you. Imagine yourself as either hand or flame; your "opponent" as the other; your conversation as movement.

Find the path of gentility and harmony in between words and gestures. Stay in it, soft and open—completely alert, forgetting everything you have ever felt about this person, bringing nothing but your awareness with you, expecting nothing, judging nothing, wanting nothing. The objective is to enter the energy field you create together. Use it to *know* the other person. Wait for truth to surface. When it does, respond directly. Respond with compassion.

Work on bringing this knowledge into your daily relationships.

Resolutions
Being the Flame; Being the Hand

✧ Today, instead of creating resistance, I will surrender to the life force within me. I will trust and follow it into harmony with others.

✧ Today, I will remember that when I am in harmony, I am safe.

✧ Today, I will not impose my values and conclusions on those I wish to know.

✧ Today, I will attentively observe and listen to those with whom I am in contact.

✧ Today, I will let go of doubt and let my feelings and intuitions guide me to where I should be.

✧ Today, I will look for opportunities to better know those I already think I know.

✧ Today, I will not condemn or condone anyone freely expressing who they are.

✧ Today, I will actively respect the sentiments of others, even though I may disagree with them.

✧ Today, I will remember that my silence lacks only one thing: the sound of my voice.

✧ Today, I will not demand anything. I will problem-solve by using only perception.

4
Assessing Threats
Conquer Your Fear

*Stop talking, stop thinking,
and there is nothing
you will not understand.*

—SENG-TS'AN

Although we cannot stop pain from entering our lives, we can control our response to it. Most martial artists learn early on that the first step in dealing with pain is to distinguish a real threat from a nonthreat. The first time I learned to differentiate between the two was the first time I saw a kick coming right for my head. My reaction must have been a sight. I completely froze in anticipation of getting hit—so much so that I couldn't have done anything to avoid the kick, even if I'd wanted to. Needless to say, I got punched in the ribs.

I relived similar scenarios during the next few classes. Finally my instructor, watching me take one hit after another, had a talk with me.

"Most of the kicks that immobilized you," he explained, "wouldn't have reached you in the first place. They were being fired from too far away." He explained that like many new students, I was still having trouble conquering my fear. To do so, I must first assess the threat. He told me to imagine a circle around me—of any color. The circle should be longer than the length of one of his kicks, a distance large enough to put me out of harm's way. Then he told me to imagine another circle, of a different color, a little longer than the length of a punch. These were my ranges.

"If an opponent enters them, you should consider his or her actions a threat and decide on an appropriate response."

I could block, counterattack, retreat, or any combination of these—anything that was appropriate within those ranges. If, however, opponents remained outside my circles, they could make all the noise they wanted, throw any kind of strike, taunt me, whatever, but *I was to stay calm*; they would be of no threat.

But nonthreats work. One of the most basic sparring strategies a martial artist learns is how to use a *feint*, or decoy. We love them. We throw a strike, a punch, or a kick, which our opponent will perceive as a threat. While our opponent is paying attention to that, we throw the one that really matters. All martial artists do this. Why? Because it works—even on the most experienced.

Here's an example: One day, another student and I

were sparring. We got in close, and he suddenly jetted both arms forward, wide open, as though he was going to tag me with the ridge of his hands, on both respective sides of my head simultaneously. When I went chasing after the strikes, he immediately pulled his arms in and came at me with a flurry of *straight* punches, as if he were doing the fifty-yard dash down my center. Despite the fact that his feint was huge and—you'd think—obvious, it had worked. I just couldn't believe I'd chased such a thing. Even after I became aware of the decoy, he was still able to pull it off. I remember thinking that moves like that could only work on novices. So I tried the same feint on a veteran student, and to my surprise, and his, it worked. Assessing threats is always difficult and something we constantly need to work on. The trick is to conquer our fear.

My instructor had several drills that were intended to help clear out unnecessary fears and hold our focus on what was important. Once, he pulled out a pair of enormous, fourteen-pound boxing gloves—four to five times the size of a normal fist. He paired me up with a partner and told me to hold my hands behind my back. We were to stand toe-to-toe, and my partner, who was given the gloves, was to launch strikes at my head, using about 75 percent of his normal force. I was supposed to be learning something about bobbing back and forth and getting away from my partner's strikes (and by the way, my partner had been told that he was next).

Our teacher, seeing the look in our eyes, took back the gloves and told us he was going to take a few shots at each of us at about 25 percent torque. I remember how even a strike that light concerned me, but when it hit, I realized it was nothing. It felt like getting hit with a small pillow. Threat was gone, and with it my fear.

Getting rid of fear helps us focus on the right things. Once my partner and I abandoned the fear of getting hit, we were able to concentrate on the important element of the drill, which was on building up the necessary movements and confidence to *dodge* oncoming strikes. What at first had made me anxious turned out to be one of my favorite exercises. To this day, I use it to further hone my sparring skills and to help condition unnecessary fears away.

Of course, "conquer your fear" is easier said than done. Sometimes a threat is real, and it is certainly painful. On these occasions, I have found calming devices such as mushin and regulated breathing effective ways of lowering the pain; and in some cases, focused, directed chi is a good way to prevent or eliminate pain. I'm not suggesting that this is an easy or overnight fix, but rather a pattern of techniques that require practice and integration into our lives in order to reap their many benefits.

Recently I found an occasion to utilize these skills during a laparoscopic abdominal operation. My imagination was getting the best of me, and I began to fear all kinds of unknown things about surgery. I tried to focus on reasons why the procedure wasn't threatening. It was elective on my part, and while there *were* issues of pain and recovery, they would be minimal and manageable. Besides, the doctor was confident the surgery would be successful, which meant the elimination of a discomfort I'd been walking around with for months.

When the time came, however, I was still apprehensive. I tried to keep my mind clear of emotion and forced my concentration to a diagram on the wall. Even though I couldn't read it from where I was positioned, it was enough to keep my mind off what was happening and minimize my anxieties. I regulated my breathing and tried to stay calm, and in the end, I managed to transport myself from harm's way until I heard the doctor remarking, "Now, that wasn't so bad, was it?"

I had lost track of time and was amazed the operation was over. "No," I said. "It wasn't."

Whenever you use these skills to help transcend a daunting situation, you will walk away revitalized. You will have pride and confidence in your power to protect yourself. You will feel freer. You will be more content. You will live more heartily, experience more, and accomplish more.

You can control your response to pain. Practice assessing threats. Conquer your fear. Use your skills to respond to real threats and help dismiss nonthreats. Stay calm. Be flexible. Flood yourself with positive energy. Trust in yourself.

Meditation
Assessing Threats

Avoid entangled thoughts,
that you may see the explanation
in Paradise.

—Divni Shâmsi Tabrizâ

Consider a situation that is bringing pain—physical, emotional, spiritual—into your life. Identify the times and places where it occurs. Close your eyes and visualize character(s) and events, from your own point of view, or objectively, looking from outside in (in this case, you become one of the characters, and you can watch yourself from a variety of vantage points: from behind, above, below, in front, and so on). You can also observe the action from anybody or anything else in the picture's perspective. I encourage exploring multiple points of view.

Consider all the details within the picture and differentiate between real threats and nonthreats. Dismiss the nonthreats. Make a statement to yourself telling yourself that they have no power over you.

Shift your attention to something in your environment that you perceive as nonthreatening, if you must, to help you refocus. Use it to help calm and center you. Summon your chi to give you strength and protect you.

Revitalize yourself. Let a feeling of love and power flow within you.

Ask your inner self what special tools you need to deal with whatever threats have manifested themselves. Do you require softness, gentility, wisdom, thankfulness, compassion, joy, empathy, goodwill, humor, strength? Imagine someone you know who has the qualities needed to dissolve these threats admirably. Place that person in your situation. When we open ourselves to others and their gifts, we create the possibility of receiving those gifts. How would the person you have selected respond? What special tools does he or she have that would make a response successful? Add those tools to the ones you have already identified would be needed and simply summon them all. Feel them coming to you. Make yourself attentive, and wait until the exact moment to use them opens itself to you.

Resolutions
Assessing Threats

✧ Today, I will actively and attentively remember that I am free to choose my reactions to challenges.

✧ Today, I will try to remain calm and flexible in my attempts to differentiate threat from nonthreat.

✧ Today, I will look for opportunities to identify and dismiss nonthreatening situations.

✧ Today, I will approach the day's events without fear.

✧ Today, I will invoke the power of the Infinite into my mind, body, and spirit, and I will surrender myself to its abundance.

✧ Today, I will surrender myself to the love and power that I am. And for this I will be grateful.

5
Seeing with Your Skin
Develop Your Sensitivity and Intuition

Forget all about brush and ink.
Then you will know the beauty
of landscapes.

—CHING HAO

Sensitivity is a major concept in martial arts training. One of my instructor's favorite phrases is *See with your skin.*

"Sensitivity," he would say, "is a key that will unlock many doors."

The word *sensitivity* itself can be traced to the Latin *sens*, meaning "to feel." It can be defined as "understanding something well enough to act on it." In its noun form, it can refer to someone with psychic powers. Sensitivity may best be understood simply as intuition.

Sensitivity is natural, and it is essential. In many ways, it is a language unto itself. Just think of all you can say to someone, at times, with a simple pat on the shoulder.

How many words would it take to explain all you can feel and share in such an instant?

I remember when my instructor first introduced the concept of sensitivity into our training—how intrigued I was that something like the ability to *feel* had to be relearned.

"Focus on your feet," he said. "What do you feel beneath them?"

"The floor," I answered.

"Close your eyes. Eyes can be deceptive," he asserted. "You have to learn how to see with your skin."

I closed my eyes. After a few moments of silence, I added, "I can feel the bottoms of my feet, the air surrounding them, and the blood flowing through them."

"That's good. Now make yourself feel more. What else can you feel?"

"My skin and muscle," I said.

"What more?"

"My legs, hips, weight, the rest of my body—torso, shoulders, arms, hands, head, my breath, you—I have some sense of you," I added. "And the building and the various machines in the building, the energy below it and above it, the breeze coming in through the window."

"That's it," he said.

Seeing with your skin means to use more than just your eyes to observe and listen to others. You can sense (*sens*) with deeper perception and consciousness. Use all of you. The more you can feel, the better you will be at determining how and when to react to an opponent—or *if* you need to react at all. Sensitivity will quicken your mind and develop your intuition.

The instructor asked me to stand a few inches away from him. This time, he closed *his* eyes and placed a hand on my chest, instructing me to take a shot at him. I threw a high strike, and he met it with an immediate block. There was that uncanny ability of his to read my mind again.

"Throw any kind of strike you want," he said.

It didn't matter if I kicked, punched, or reached to grab, he was right there blocking and countering.

"Once you make contact with an opponent, you should be able to sense what his or her next move will be," he emphasized.

There are two types of sensitivity, internal and external: yin and yang. Yin (internal) is connected with our mysterious powers of intuition, while yang (external) is connected with our powers of reason. Yin is the energy in the Universe that is reproductive and creative, whereas yang is productive and rational.

Seeing with our skin is, in essence, shifting our attention inward, where responses do not rely on net muscular strength, but rather on a keen awareness of chi. This shift is essential in quickening our ability to sense another's movements. At the precise point at which we intuit a movement and then act upon that knowledge, we are shifting our attention from yin to yang or from the internal to the external—and thus are maintaining a harmonious flow of energy in our actions and throughout our lives.

Making ourselves aware of this shift in attention and practicing it regularly helps strengthen sensitivity and intuition and gives it a say in what we do. We begin to move more fluidly. We are able to find better balance with others and the world around us. We connect with others more often. Our mind quickens and experiences deepen.

At first, I used to think we trained with sensitivity drills simply to improve speed and accuracy. Although that *was* part of it, little did I know that the exercises were ultimately designed to help us transcend the sensory limitations of our bodies.

One of the most traditional and more advanced sensitivity drills we trained with was the Kung Fu exercise known as *chi sao* (clinging arms). Our objective was to position our arms and hands as though we were holding a soccer ball about a foot in front of our chests. Then we stood toe-to-toe, our arms and hands maintaining the same posture, and touched forearms. From there, we each gently pushed our imaginary soccer ball forward toward the center of each other's chest, giving the ball a half turn (left–right, right–left, and so on) as we continued the drill. The point was to maintain contact with our partner's arms and to make ourselves ultrasensitive to each other's energy. We had to focus our attention inward and try to intuit each other's slightest movement. We were told to look for openings between our partner's hands or arms and to take shots if we found them.

The drill was not competitive but rather intended to heighten our ability to feel each other's chi and to intuit what direction it was headed. Hence the sensation of knowing what a partner is going to do before he or she does it. We could then block the action, move with it, or strike.

Sensitivity and intuition require softness and calm—otherwise we may not be able to tune in to them. We have to stay loose, unassuming, and acutely present.

As I recall the various partners I worked chi sao with, one stands out. He was a hulk of a man, weighing well over three hundred pounds. Everyone wanted to experience what it was like to work with such a giant. Ironically, his approach was so light that you thought you could strike through his arms with the slightest force. And when you tried, an acute awareness would flare through them, and they would snap like a whip, redirecting wherever you were headed, knocking you off balance, and ultimately overcoming you. He never relied on muscular strength. His power came from within.

Sensitivity and intuition are natural. Off the mats we

have all experienced the ability to know something before it actually occurs. For many of us, this happens when we bump into a person we haven't seen or heard from in a long time, often in close proximity to when we've been thinking about him or her.

Here are a few other examples: Having played the violin for years, I've experienced many incidents in which someone intuitively felt an opening in the music and slipped into a moment's improvisation, dazzling everyone with how beautifully (and perfectly) the unexpected riff fit—so much so, in fact, that anyone unfamiliar with the piece could hardly believe it wasn't scripted. To the musician, acting purely from sensitivity and intuition (*feeling*, as they say), the movement seemed completely natural.

Public speaking and interpersonal conversations work similarly. Many times, when addressing an audience, we choose to stop short of lines that appear in the text because the moment makes it appropriate to do so. Other times, we add to what's there. We know it's right when we feel we've connected with someone. We use these skills in everyday conversation, as well, adding to what we would normally say in a particular situation or, at times, cutting ourselves off. When we connect, we know it. We feel exhilarated.

Sensitivity and intuition help us know when to make a move and how to fit in to where we want to be. They help keep us from being manipulated. We become better communicators and partners in all our relations. Sensitivity and intuition can help keep us safe. They can help guide us toward our goals, especially in moments of confusion. Moreover, they can guide us to our innermost self. The more we develop these skills, the more we experience their rewards, the more committed we will become to making their cultivation a lifelong process.

Go inward where the mind is free and infinite. Practice seeing with your skin. Instead of simply having "thoughts," learn "being" your mind. Trust your instincts. Live serenely and purely. Live freely. Fit in.

Meditation
Seeing with Your Skin

*There is power in sight which is superior
to the eyes set in the head
and more far-reaching
than the heavens and the earth.*
— MEISTER ECKHART

The following meditation is based on chi sao. In order to practice it appropriately, you will need a partner.

Stand facing each other. Center and breathe slowly. Relax your whole body. Follow your breath in, shifting your awareness down to your Lower Dan Tien. Feel the cleansing and nourishing effect of your breathing with each breath. Empty your mind. Feel the heightened energy of your chi as you breathe. Visualize your brightened chi flowing outward, surrounding your body with protective and nourishing energy (I like to visualize this as healing white light). *Make your body as supple as possible* so that it releases any tension that may block you from feeling another's energy.

One-Handed Chi Sao

Position I. You and your partner should position yourselves face-to-face and close enough to touch each other's foreheads with the palms of your right hands.

Once you establish this distance, let your arms return loosely to your sides.

Begin by extending your right arm and bending it upward, forming a near ninety-degree angle and keeping your hand open in a prayer position. Likewise, your partner should place his or her left arm so that it crosses the "outside" of your arm, forming an X between you. The inside of your partner's forearm should be touching against the outside of your own. Both of you should keep your hands open in a prayer position. Relax. Stay as loose as possible. Make your arms light as air.

Position 2. Softly and lightly move your right arm slightly *forward and backward* (maintaining adhesion) toward your partner's centerline (the imaginary line coming down the front of his or her body). *Important: Your upper arm directs the movement.* Your forearm is more or less stationary, like a hinge.

Both of you should allow your wrists to remain flexible as you rotate, gliding each other's movement. When you do this, your wrist works like a roller, more smoothly gliding your partner's arm back and forth.

Your job is to aim the outside blade of your prayer hand at the center of your partner's chest. Keep your movement slow and fluid. Your partner's job is to maintain adhesion, stay ultrasoft and light, and harmoniously glide with your own hand as it approaches.

The point is to glide with each other.

Continue this movement, both of you cooperating

with each other, until you feel you have it down. You will establish a rhythm. You will feel the adhesion and rotation of your wrists, each of you supporting the other.

Stay with it. If you think you're overextending your arm, move closer to your partner.

Note: Your other hand should remain loose at your side throughout the exercise.

Stay centered. Try to feel your chi moving through your arms and feel as much of your partner's energy as possible.

Repeat Position 2 several times, making yourself sensitive to your partner's energy and how yours flows with it. *Use all of "you" to observe and listen to each other.*

Now you are ready to further develop your skills of sensitivity and intuition.

For Position 3, designate one of you as the aggressor, the other as defender. It's better to trade off—one shot each for a while. When you get used to the exercise, you can do the drill without identifying an aggressor and defender. You can just let things progress naturally.

Ideally, when this part of the drill is being done by two masters, neither gets any strikes on the other. Both partners have that much sensitivity, intuition, and ability to "fit in" with the other's movement. That's what you're striving for.

Position 3. Continue the back-and-forth arm movement. If you are the designated agressor and you intuit an opportunity, you should attempt to touch (very lightly) your partner's forehead (or center chest) with the palm of your hand.

Keep your movements slow. Do *not* increase speed in order to get the shot in. Maintain the same speed you have established in the exercise. The idea here is to use your sensitivity and intuition to find openings in your partner's movement, at which time you can take your shot (if you are the aggressor), or to identify and protect your vulnerabilities during incoming shots and still maintain harmony with your partner (if you are the defender).

The defending partner should not block the first half dozen or so incoming shots. Let your partner have them so that you can both see and feel how the exercise works.

Then, after you get the idea, start trying to stop the incoming strikes, using your hand, primarily (as in Position 2), to simply guide or glide the shot away from you. *You will have to concentrate on not allowing yourself to get jumpy and speed up or harden your responses.*

Switch roles. You will discover many ways to find openings in each other's movements, as well as to protect your own vulnerabilities, yet stay in harmony the entire time.

Remember, your job is to always maintain adhesion with your partner.

Advanced version. Either of you can try maintaining the aforementioned positions, moving your arms or wrists in small circular (clockwise) patterns, rather than coming straight forward, again maintaining adhesion.

Don't fight the movement. Stay ultrasoft. Harmonize. For more of a challenge, try moving counterclockwise as well.

You can also try extending, even straightening, your forearm and moving your whole arm in larger circular motions, blending these with smaller circles. Try bringing your arm downward and then breaking into a circular pattern. Or bring it upward, or what have you. You can make circles with your whole arm or tiny ones with your wrist. Each opens different possibilities.

Patience is a must. Don't initiate a shot unless you feel or intuit an opening.

After you have practiced one-handed chi sao this way for a while, you can work it so that there is no designated aggressor or defender. You can both take shots whenever you feel the possibility. I encourage you to try this with many partners. This will help you develop your sensitivity and intuition based on a variety of different people's expressions of their own.

To further train these skills and heighten your sensitivity, try chi sao blindfolded.

Chi sao demonstrates that we can fully express ourselves and, at the same time, fit in—that is, exist in harmony with others—by using sensitivity and intuition.

Reflect on ways you can transfer these skills into everyday life in order to improve self-awareness, trust, communication, intimacy, spontaneity, and many other aspects of your life. Then try them out in your daily relationships.

Resolutions
Seeing with Your Skin

✧ Today, if I catch myself trying to control what I see, I will detach and put as much energy into increasing my sensitivity in conversations as I would into trying to control them.

✧ Today, I will practice trusting my intuition, allowing myself to understand and know in a more primal way.

✧ Today, I will try observing and listening more than I speak, and I will allow my feelings to inform me when I do speak.

✧ Today, I will stop trying to make things happen.

✧ Today, I will stop overextending myself.

✧ Today, I will listen to the voice of my spirit and let it guide me toward happiness.

✧ Today, I will trust in the power of the Infinite to inform me as it moves in and through all life—both people and situations.

6
Knowing Your Targets

Control Your Urges

Truth comes in between breaths.
—BUDDHA

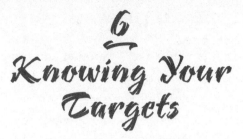y teacher once told me, "You don't have to take a breath with every single movement." He was speaking literally in regard to a kata I was performing. *Katas* are martial arts forms that look like dances.

We were working a series of movements in coordination with regulated breathing. He was explaining how slow, deep breathing intensifies attentiveness in meditation and strength in form and combat. Metaphorically, though, he was referencing much more. Still, any conclusions there were to be drawn from his analogy had been left for me to discover on my own. That was his way.

The first thing I found out was that not breathing for every movement forced my mind to remain focused—it became harder to let thoughts stray.

But I soon discovered another meaning to my teacher's words. I was a novice and sparring with an opponent who had a few months' experience on me. I'd already figured out that *truth-coming-between-breaths* was a sort of combat strategy—that an "opening," or vulnerability in my opponent, would manifest itself if I controlled my urges to hit where I wanted to hit and actively waited; if I simply surrendered myself to the flow of the match.

So there I was, going with the flow, so to speak—trying to practice what my instructor had taught me—and instead of looking good with my new strategy, I got tagged, not once but several times.

My teacher just looked at me with an *oh-well* expression that let me know it was merely a matter of time before I mastered this lesson. He was right. I soon figured out that I was losing because I was *thinking* about how to apply what he had told me. In martial arts, as in life, you quickly learn not to think too much. You have to *do*. While you're thinking, you open spaces where an opponent can successfully strike at you. The more you think, the more vulnerable you become. But controlling urges isn't easy. I gave myself room to stumble until one day it happened. I wasn't thinking, just moving, when my sparring partner opened up, and there it was, right in front of me, big as a billboard: an enormous, open target. I took my shot and landed the strike. It all happened smoothly and automatically.

Little by little, you begin to trust the process, and it gets easier. In time, your responses quicken and become more effortless.

You learn that the targets you're looking for come in between what you think is going to happen (or think you can make happen) and your opponent's actions. You learn that the truth of any moment comes in between the breath of your thoughts. You learn to remain calm and attentive, and equally as important, you learn the virtues of controlling your urges, of waiting for the right moment before taking action. Sometimes you need to get out of your own way in order to see the real targets. Then you learn to go at them swiftly and directly and with the appropriate force to hit the bull's-eye.

These skills transfer into life situations on a daily basis. For me, it happened one fall at the college where I teach. I had decided to apply for a sabbatical during the spring semester of the following school year. This meant that I had to have a plan for what I was going to do during my time off, and it had to be approved.

I was anxious to get everything done, and before long it seemed I was spending every waking hour thinking or talking about my sabbatical. As I became more anxious, so did everyone around me. You know the situation: After a while, you've said all there is to say, and you still don't have the answer—you're only mulling over what's already been said, and you know that's not good enough. Frustrated and pressured as the date for the application approached, I told myself to put my martial arts skills to work and simply forget about the issue; resolution would come. I had to control my urges and wait. I assured myself that truth would come.

Then, of course, the answer surfaced when I least expected it to—all on its own.

My wife and I were out hiking an Adirondack trail when suddenly, out of nowhere, the answer flashed before me. I told her about it right there on the trail. We both knew that it was right, and the approval committee agreed, because a few weeks later my sabbatical was granted.

All the smaller (but often more taxing) hassles of life resolve in the same way. You are having a family disagreement that goes on for months. You torture yourself looking for a way out of the problem. You try things to resolve the issue even though your heart tells you it wouldn't be happy with such a solution. You don't listen to yourself and make yourself even more miserable. Then one day you're in the shower. You're not thinking about anything, not even washing. You are in what we all refer to as automatic pilot. And suddenly, out of nowhere, the answer flashes at you—"big as a billboard." Every cell of you knows it's the right answer, too. You use it. It works.

Accept this pattern. Learn from it. You will save yourself all kinds of time and heartache. You will waste fewer days beating yourself up looking for solutions to problems before the answers are about to give themselves to you. And perhaps there is a reason for the wait. For in waiting, we learn.

Life is constantly demanding solutions to one thing or another. Nevertheless, stay calm, control your urges, and actively wait: Go for a jog, take a drive, chop wood, listen to music, wash and put away dishes, sweep a floor—anything you can do to slowly get your mind off the urgency. If you have to, act as though you have already taken care of the problem, until you actually do—just to get your mind off it.

Be attentive. You will be amazed at how easily solutions can come.

Waiting isn't easy, but acting when the time isn't right can make us vulnerable and further our distance from what we are trying to achieve. We don't have to judge or justify. We can make a conscious decision to simply act as if all will be fine as we wait for life's openings to manifest. Our job is to control the urge to strike—until the target is right, to live attentively, enjoy our lives, and wait for the right moment. Truth will come.

Meditation
Knowing Your Targets

Where every "where" and
every "when" is focused.
           —DANTE

Consider the last time you attempted to make something happen before it was ready to occur naturally and on its own. How would the opening have manifested itself to you had you waited? What constructive (energy-building and strengthening) things could have been done with your time as you waited? What steps could you have taken to slow yourself down and prepare yourself to achieve the goal when it offered itself to you?

Think back to the last time waiting helped you to see more. What were the virtues of having waited? Can you identify the stages you experienced as you actively waited? Could your strategy, at any given point, have been enhanced?

Resolutions
Knowing Your Targets

✧ Today, I will be open to the truth.

✧ Today, I will remain attentive as I wait for the truth.

✧ Today, I will remain centered and relaxed.

✧ Today, I will trust that there is a plan for me and that I am being prepared for the journey.

✧ Today, I will be confident that my tools will enable me to gather the truth as it reveals itself to me.

✧ Today, I will give myself permission to stumble and learn from my mistakes as I seek the truth.

✧ Today, I will give myself permission to slow down as I seek the truth.

✧ Today, I will practice skipping a beat in conversations, pausing to better be present for the truth.

✧ Today, I will speak the truth, and I will speak it when the time is right, not before or after.

✧ Today, I will welcome the truth, and I will remember that truth is connected to the Infinite from which all love, peace, and power come, and I will feel abundant strength and rootedness.

✧ Today, I will be thankful for what I see.

7
Intensifying Your Effort and Striking
Channel Your Energy

Flexibility masters hardness.
—Jiu Yoku Go O Sei Uuru

ll martial artists are interested in finding ways to intensify the power of their techniques—and at the same time not get hurt by the backlash. Sound familiar? Probably. You don't have to be a martial artist to want to make your moves from a point of strength and avoid negative repercussions.

Pulling away in martial arts refers to the retraction of strikes. At a basic level, students learn to pull back a shot primarily so that it doesn't "hang out there" and become a target for their opponent, and also so that it can be used again if necessary.

A big part of martial arts training is learning how to

channel your energy. At some point, you learn that there are other, perhaps less obvious, reasons for pulling away. These other reasons have to do with issuing power or, more precisely, with the transfer of close-range, explosive power known as *cun jing* (inch power) into a target without being harmed by the recoil of energy.

The martial arts are loaded with stories about this coveted ability, and we love to tell them. One such story is of a martial arts master who, with one close-range strike, could break a single brick placed midway in a stack of bricks three feet high. The energy could be transferred with that level of extreme power and precision.

Some of my fellow students had sworn they had seen this technique performed and that there was no apparent gimmick involved. I, on the other hand, had never seen anyone perform such a feat, but was enthralled by the wonderful trails of exploration it suggested.

There is support for ideas of energy transfer outside the world of martial arts. A good example of this comes from the teachings of the late philosopher-theologian Joseph Campbell, who defined consciousness as something that does not exist in the head (or mind), but rather is directed by the mind. "Consciousness and energy," said Campbell, "are perhaps the same thing." Thus, when we direct our energy, we are also directing our consciousness, and vice versa.

Martial arts' most colorful and best-known example of directing cun jing was brought into the limelight by Bruce Lee with his legendary one-inch punch. Lee was able to dazzle spectators with devastating power unleashed from within an inch of a target—be it wood or an opponent. Of course, nearly everyone studying martial arts wants to know how Bruce Lee did it.

To demonstrate the mechanics of the technique, my teacher gathered a handful of phone books and handed me three of them. "These are to protect you," he said.

He told me to hold the phone books flat against my abdomen like a shield.

"You won't get hurt," he assured me. "The phone books will absorb most of the shock."

Then, from no more than an inch away, he launched a quick punch that, after contact, he retracted almost instantly. For a second, I felt only the thrust of the shot—and then, a curious swell of energy about the size of a golf ball moving through my abdomen. It was uncanny. It felt as if at any moment the amassed energy inside me could explode into pain. But it never did, and what's more, there were no marks anywhere. It was as though the energy had been injected into me and passed straight through my body.

Later, my teacher explained that what I had felt was a transfer of his energy passing through me, and that if I hadn't had the phone books to absorb some of it, I could have been seriously injured. That kind of strike can pass straight through someone, cause little damage to the area of immediate contact, hardly moving the person at all, yet leaving a bruise on his or her back.

"There are three key factors to making the technique work," he added. "First, relax. Then, put your whole body into it. Lastly, you have to develop two speeds: a forward thrust and a retraction. *Both* are equally important."

He demonstrated the punch on a heavy bag and then on a cinder-block wall. I was amazed at how hard he could strike the cinder blocks without any damage to his hand. When I'd attempted to strike the same wall, at a tenth the velocity, I'd come close to breaking my knuckles because I had the forward thrust, but not the pullback.

With a much quicker retraction, I would have been able to deliver more energy into the target, yet spare myself the pain of my own energy recoiling back at me.

We began to train staying loose, putting all of our relaxing and centering techniques together before attempting to issue a strike. You can't be tight at all when trying to generate power from this short distance. The softer you remain, the less tension your muscles hold, the faster you can move.

We had to start learning how to condense our chi and channel it to generate the power we were after.

This sounds complicated, but it doesn't have to be. We worked the basic adage, *Wherever the mind goes, your chi goes.*

Accordingly, we trained directing chi by visualizing it moving in sync with our breathing. With our in-breaths we visualized drawing chi from our extremities to the center of our body, condensing it tightly into a smaller and smaller space (like sunlight tightened into a dot by a magnifying lens). Then we channeled its concentrated form back into our arms and hands, feet and legs with our out-breaths. This technique of using breath and mind to direct the flow of chi greatly intensified our issuance of power.

Little by little, we learned how to stay more softly focused, channel energy to those parts of our body that needed it to deliver a technique, and build up the power we needed to execute and retract a shot powerfully and without harm to ourselves.

We all have the need to channel our energy from time to time. Deadlines nearly always require an intense effort, at some point, in order to get the job done. Not long ago, I was completing the final edits on a paper I was to present at a conference when, all of a sudden, my computer bombed. Despite several attempts to fix it, I slowly realized that the manuscript I'd been working on was irretrievable.

I couldn't believe it—the text was more than forty pages in length, and I hadn't backed up any of the work in nearly a week. There were no recent hard copies.

Needless to say, I started to panic. I thought about the nonrefundable airline tickets. I thought about the irretrievable text. My thoughts raced from all my complaints against unresolved kinks in my computer software to what was I going to do about the presentation—it was less than twenty-four hours away.

I became angry and then fearful and wasted nearly half an hour in this agitated mode. I allowed myself to feel what I was feeling. But I knew that I was going to have to shift gears. I wasn't getting anywhere and was losing time.

I took a few deep breaths. I told myself that although things didn't look great, they weren't really as disastrous as I had originally believed. Tension of any sort gets into the muscles and the mind. It slows us down and restricts movement.

I remembered that somewhere in the office there were handwritten sketches with most of that week's writing. They would be a good start toward reassembling the lost text. The more I calmed and faced the situation, the more a solution began to materialize—and, in return, the more relaxed I became. The effect was synergistic.

Then as with so many other times in life when I needed immediate strength, I told myself that somehow everything would work out. Given this opportunity to go at it a second time, I would write the paper even better.

I summoned and condensed as much energy as possible, channeled streams of clean positive energy everywhere I needed it, and went on to the task of retyping. In addition,

I promised myself that when I finished, I would immediately shift (pull away) from the job and treat myself to a dinner at a good restaurant with my wife—no matter what the time. That was my manner of pulling away from the intense expenditure of energy. There are many tactics for pulling away—physical, verbal, situational, emotional, spiritual, and so on. Which you choose is determined by the particulars of your situation. But as the concept goes, you cannot output large amounts of energy *without* pulling back. The risk of recoil is too great.

As for me, I rewrote the paper and would like to believe that it did turn out better in its revised form. My wife and I had a wonderfully satisfying dinner that evening. I felt good, and the shift helped lighten my spirits and regenerate my excitement over the presentation I would be giving. I woke up the next day feeling restored and free of conflict.

Life is full of situations that require quick and intense force. You can learn to deal with them powerfully and avoid potential backlash. Relax, heighten your attention, and stay in the moment. Practice intensifying your effort. Channel your energy. Take your shot, and remember to pull away.

Meditation
Intensifying Your Effort and Striking

See first with your mind,
then with your eyes,
and finally with your body.
— YAGYU MUNENORI

This meditation is designed to help you experience (feel) and coordinate each stage of generating inch power and pulling away.

In actual everyday practice, the process of energy building and transfer can be internal, requiring no external movement at all.

What is important is to transfer the concept of focused energy and breath into your daily life and begin to use it to live more effectively and dynamically.

Read through the stages first so that you have a basic understanding of what is required. Then give them a try.

Have patience. It may take you several attempts before you can smoothly maneuver through the postures. Concentration is very important, for there are many distracters—including your own self-awareness. Nonetheless, try to maintain a steady focus.

Note: Perform this meditation in a standing position.

Stage 1. Blue: Relax. Stand naturally with your arms hanging loose at your sides. Place your right foot forward (about twelve inches) and let your energy sink downward. Simultaneously, bend your knees a little. Visualize yourself standing in the center of a circle that extends about three feet in diameter. Imagine the area within the circle as calming blue.

Center. Breathe slowly and smoothly. Inhale through your nose and exhale through your mouth. When you feel relaxed, breathe more deeply to a brisk ten-count. If a count of ten is too strenuous, try five or less until you can work your way up.

Follow your breath to your Lower Dan Tien. Hold your breath there, also for a brisk ten-count, then slowly release it.

Stage 2. Green: Gather energy. Continue deep breathing. Step forward with your left foot, two steps, leaving your right foot as the lead both times. Again, sink your energy downward and assume the same stance as in Stage 1.

Visualize yourself at the center of a circle exactly as in Stage 1, only this time make it green.

Then visualize yourself drawing chi from all your limbs with your in-breath. Let it gather in Lower Dan Tien.

Stage 3. Yellow: Condense energy. Continue deep breathing. Step forward (right foot lead) into another circle, this time a yellow one.

With each in-breath, continue drawing energy from every cell in your body and sinking it downward.

Visualize condensing and storing your chi into a smaller space, compressing the space more and more with each breath. Feel your energy building up as you draw and compress more chi.

Stage 4. Bright red: Direct energy. Continue deep breathing. Step forward, keeping all the same postures as previously, and enter one last circle, a bright red one. Your energy should be abundant.

Enter this space with the understanding that you are going to release the energy that you have built up.

Condense your chi one more time, drawing from your whole body, from the earth, and from the heavens, condensing it maximally.

Then, with your out-breath, direct your chi forward to the lower outside corner of your right hand and extend it slowly forward (palm out), smoothly, effortlessly, as though your forearm were floating on water. Let yourself feel the concentrated energy flowing into a space about the size of a fifty-cent piece, in the lower right corner of your palm. Direct all of your energy there.

Do not fully straighten your arm.

Imagine a wall about one foot away. Stop when your lower palm (where energy has been directed) would first make contact with the wall.

Stage 5. Working back through the cycle: Red, Yellow, Green, Blue. Relax your breathing. Discontinue condensing chi and begin to slowly retract your forearm, *mentally* working your way back (through the color circles) to the state of calm attention, where your meditation began.

Try to keep everything in sync, so that when your arms are again at your sides, you are imagining your blue circle again.

Remember, you can't stay in a red zone (intense moment) forever. You have to return to the blue (relaxed posture). Such is the cycle of yin-yang.

Repeat this meditation several times. Try moving from blue to red with fewer breaths.

Advanced version. Stand *stationary* and visualize the color of your circle changing from blue to green, yellow, and red.

Try going from Stage 1 to Stage 5 (pulling away) in an instant.

The transfer of energy should feel like bouncing a soccer ball back and forth off the wall at close range. Be sure not to overextend your arm.

More advanced version. Try working the cycle without the use of color.

Resolutions
Intensifying Your Effort and Striking

✧ Today, I will relax myself during stressful situations.

✧ Today, I will practice using precision in selecting those things to which I shall respond.

✧ Today, I will practice condensing my energy and channeling it specifically to where it is needed in order to better achieve my purposes.

✧ Today, I will minimize backlash, practicing pulling away and calming after expenditures of energy.

8
Feeling the Rhythm
Respond Appropriately

Do not permit the events of your daily lives to bind you,
but never withdraw yourselves from them.
Only by acting thus can you earn the title
"A Liberated One."

—HUANG PO

All martial arts emphasize that good rhythm is essential for responding appropriately to any given situation. Developing a high sensitivity to your internal rhythms, as well as the rhythms of others, will create many opportunities in everyday life, just as it does on the mats.

By definition, *rhythm* refers to patterns, and life is a series of patterns. Thus, all of life is rhythmic. Good rhythm helps us move more naturally and effectively toward what we are attempting to accomplish and with whom, by putting us in sync with other movement in our environment. It helps us create and take advantage of life's openings, as well as protecting ourselves against vulnerabilities. It can overcome inequities in size and power.

Rhythm exercises became an integral part of my martial arts training. One drill was called *hubud*. These are partnered arm-to-arm exercises in which one partner throws a specific strike and the other blocks it and returns the same strike with his or her blocking arm. In turn, this allows the first partner to respond with the same pattern of blocking, sweeping, and striking.

What's important is getting in touch with your own, as well as your opponent's, rhythms—when they're alike, when they're different, and especially when and how you can alter them. This isn't so hard. Our basic pattern was based on the movement: 1 (block), 2 (sweep), 3 (punch). To keep us focused, our instructor would snap his fingers on a steady downbeat as he directed us through each of the movements.

Once I became aware of the rhythm, I was able to work the drill without having to look. In fact, after a while, we practiced blindfolded. This further sensitized the harmony of our movements, as well as our intuition.

Practice paid off. After a while, I was able to get in on less experienced opponents, but I was still unable to defend or tag anyone more advanced. Experience was part of it. But, as I suspected, there were other reasons, too.

To respond appropriately, you have to know *when* to attempt to get what you want. In martial arts, this is known as *timing*. What's more, in order to know when to take your shot, you have to find an opening.

There are several ways to create openings. The primary way is simply to pay attention and identify patterns.

All of us have patterns—physical, emotional, spiritual. Perhaps you know someone whose pattern of activity just before an argument is to become quiet, then distant, then quick with responses in conversation. Conceptually, these kinds of movements aren't much different from what you look for on the mats. Identifying patterns such as these can help you divert conflict before it occurs.

But you have to be attentive. For example, although hubud is based on three movements, the same movements can be delivered in a wide variety of beats. Your partner could just as easily fit all three movements into two beats: The block and sweep could be simultaneous on the "1" count, for example, followed by the punch on "2." So to respond appropriately, you have to watch carefully. Once you recognize the pattern, though, *all you have to do is look for the spaces between beats and slip your strike in there.*

Anything that disrupts a partner's rhythm—decoys, new rhythms, strikes, and so forth—can create openings or make existing ones bigger. Your opponent basically loses focus; by the time he or she regains it, you're in.

You'll discover that the best times to use these approaches are whenever opponents are repositioning from a movement, pulling away, or beginning an attack.

At these junctures, they are committed to action; putting a cog in their intentions will generate a pause as they reassess what they are doing. This will create a space for you to respond and put the advantage on your side.

No matter if it's real life or on the mats, if you don't like the way things are going, just change the rhythm of the game and keep changing it until you create a space to respond appropriately—that is, to your advantage.

A well-known example of this is taught as streetwise self-defense—for instance, if someone is about to grab you, surprise your assailant by throwing whatever you can at him or her (even a rock) and yell, "Catch." In the moment when the attacker's attention diverts to the article, you will have a small window to make your move.

Another example occurred a while ago, when I was working with an individual who persistently trashed our colleagues. Once, when we were supposed to be working on a project, he began tongue-lashing someone I knew well. I recognized his pattern. He'd begin with his latest, Person X. Then he'd move his trashing on to supervisors, and soon the whole institution. Finally, he would flash back to an incident that occurred several years prior that had initially put him at odds with the whole place.

I decided to wait for a pause in his rant and then threw him a decoy—subtly asking him about a book he was coauthoring. The expression on his face changed from heavy to light. He took the bait and started telling me not only about the book, but also about some research he had conducted for some of its chapters. It didn't take long for him to talk himself into a more favorable state of mind. At that point, we were able to shift again and move on to issues concerning the project we were assigned.

Again, if you don't like the way things are going, just change the rhythm of the game. This is one of *my* favorite anthems.

Keep in mind that while it is important to detect and, often, to alter your opponents' rhythms, it may be advantageous to make your own rhythms less obvious and more varied. This will make it extra difficult for opponents to disrupt your actions and create openings for themselves.

Just recently, several colleagues of mine and I had designed a workshop program for a conference center up north. A few weeks prior to the conference, the center's director called to inform me that he, "according to the powers-that-be," had to visit the conference during one of the five days on which it was being held. He further told me that he was "required to evaluate the program."

"I just want to get that part of it over with as soon as time allows," he said.

He wasn't an in-your-face, up-close type of guy, but he was certainly in a rush to get this requirement behind him.

His call had caught me by surprise, and all I could

think to say at the moment was, "Sure, we'll be happy to have you there."

But he was unfamiliar with the specifics of our program, and this, combined with his attitude toward evaluation, seemed unfair. We didn't see how he could properly evaluate the conference based on one chance visit, without an overview of our objectives beforehand.

My colleagues and I wanted a good working relationship with him, but we also needed a positive and thorough evaluation in order to facilitate any future events we would participate in at the center.

That was when I got the idea that we could, perhaps, get our good evaluation—*plus* get him working with us and for us along the way.

He liked distance and left space between his phone call and his next action(s). Thus, working fast, I took advantage of the opening and lightly addressed him in his least favorite comfort zone, up close.

I broke his pattern by slipping him an email before he had a chance to get back to us. My note was formal and direct, inviting him to the first day of the conference, giving specific times and workshops to which we were welcoming him. Together, these were fully representative of the program's design and would give him what he needed for a proper evaluation.

Then I changed the patterns and tone of the game by expressing our desire to meet with him at some time prior to our conference so that we could chat about the program. That would give me and my colleagues the time we needed to present him with an overview of objectives, strategies, and procedures.

My email was tactical in that it gave him what he needed—distance. I had changed not only the pattern, but also its timing and speed. I had created the need for a quick response, which he delivered. His answer was pleasant and favorable. He thanked us for the "formal invitation" (his words) and said that he would *love* to attend our program on the day we suggested. Then he shifted (a good martial arts move on his part) and became quite cheery and personable in tone regarding the future benefits of our joint work—mine, my colleagues', and his. This new rhythm was encouraging, so I stayed with him (harmonized) and responded in kind.

Whether you are on the mats or in the middle of an everyday situation with coworkers, feeling the rhythm of the situation will help you respond appropriately.

Good rhythm will de-stress your movement, mentally and physically. You will know when and how to approach others as you work toward your goals. You will increase your confidence and chances of success. You will perceive life as more cooperative because you have learned how to cooperate with it. Many good things will come.

Identify partners' rhythms, look for (or create) your opening, and, when the time is right, make your move. Then change patterns to avoid any potential backlash.

Meditation
Feeling the Rhythm

You are not your body; you are not your brain,
not even your mind.
You are spirit.
All you have to do is reawaken to the memory,
to remember.
— BRIAN WEISS, M.D.

Consider someone you speak with on a regular basis, someone who plays a role in your daily routines. It doesn't matter what type of relationship you have with this person—formal, informal, close, relaxed, strained, what have you.

Visualize a typical conversation. Identify this individual's patterns (what he or she likes to talk about, how the person moves from one topic to another) as well as timing (when the person shifts subjects) and speed (how quickly he or she moves in conversation).

While imagining all this, try to identify any habits in your partner's body language that might signal the beginning or end of a pattern. For example, does your partner momentarily look away, pause, cross or uncross legs, eat or drink something, or the like?

Speech can also signal patterns. Does this person's

language become more emotive, more personal, or perhaps more objective and distant? Sometimes speech becomes more rapid or slows down.

Mood can also function as a prompt. Does the individual detach or become more intensely present?

Paying attention to these details can help make you aware of people's rhythms in advance of their actions, letting you divert (disrupt) or encourage (give them what they need to occur) them before they begin.

After you have successfully identified your partner's patterns, look for openings during which you can successfully enter the conversation. Consider the timing and speed of your entry so that your movement feels unstrained and natural.

Revisualize this last step and see if you could create more or larger openings by using a different timing and speed or by skipping a beat before you entered your conversation.

Now visualize yourself entering your partner's rhythms and altering them with a change in tone (formal to informal; heavier to lighter; close to distant). Consider what advantages this can provide toward your purpose. Once you are headed toward more favorable ground, shift. Stay in harmony.

You may not wish to redirect your partner's patterns. In fact, you may take pleasure in nurturing them by creating larger openings for this individual's entrance into your life. Accept the rhythm and return it in kind. Water these seeds, and you will delight in their grace.

Gently practice these skills throughout the day on the various individuals you encounter. See how you can freely move in and out of conversation and better direct it toward your goals.

Advanced version. If you feel someone is attempting to maneuver you into places you do not wish to go, try to identify that person's pattern and disrupt it before it is able to take control. The steps here are the same:

◇ Identify the pattern.

◇ Look for an opening to enter the rhythm.

◇ Respond by shifting to your own rhythm.

Try shifting to a different speed or tone as you attempt to steer things closer to where you want them to be going. You can also try the above diversion before your partner's pattern begins.

Another variation is to go into the above relation having already altered your own patterns, and maintain that change. Look for openings to appear, from which you can direct activity to more favorable places.

Resolutions
Feeling the Rhythm

✧ Today, I will be present to the people of my life and the various rhythms they employ as they work toward their aspirations.

✧ Today, I will be present to openings as they appear in the rhythms of others, and I'll use these patterns to respond appropriately.

✧ Today, I will look for opportunities to enter the rhythms of those with whom I am in conflict and redirect them toward more peaceful patterns.

✧ Today, I will look for opportunities to open myself to the rhythms of those with whom I am intimate, feeling safe inviting them in even closer, and basking in the rapture of our mutual happiness.

✧ Today, I will follow the rhythm of my joy.

2
Finding Your Range
Expand Your Comfort Zones

Those who attain the Tao . . .

*Can jump into fire
without being burned,
Walk upon reality
as if it were a void
and travel on a void
as if it were reality.
They can be at home
wherever they are.*

—T'U LUNG

n martial arts, the word *range* refers to the distance between you and your opponent or partner. There are four major ranges: kicking (measured by the length of a kick), boxing (measured by the length of a punch), trapping (toe-to-toe, close enough to trap arms), and grappling (body-to-body, close enough for takedowns). Most practitioners attempt to find their best range and excel within it. They soon find, however, that being able to float from one range to another will provide the greatest advantages and freedom on the mats—from more adaptability per situation to less predictability as an artist. Thus, one of our most critical goals is to develop proficiency in all ranges.

Whether on or off the mats, some people's modus operandi is to draw themselves close to those in their environment, while others like to maintain a distance, and still others occupy regions somewhere in between. These are the ranges in which they are most comfortable.

Our reactions to such individuals are opportunities for self-discovery. These tell us a lot about our own life ranges, especially those in which we are most and least functional. Further, they can provide us with useful information in our attempt to expand our proficiency into other ranges. This is important because proficiency in other ranges will expand our own comfort zones. We will feel freer in movement and thought. As a result, we will allow others those same freedoms. We will get more done. We will be happier people.

Martial arts ranges are based on the movements of five animals. You can have the long, sweeping, evasive speed of the crane, which likes to maintain a good distance yet can gracefully swoop to its target in an instant. Or you can have the tireless, raw, up-close, cohesive power of the tiger. You can have the fluidity of the snake or the speed of the leopard. And then there is the dragon, whose particulars I will reveal in just a few paragraphs.

The road to expanding your comfort zones is one of

discovery. Most beginners find that they already possess attributes in one of the ranges and feel comfortable when working in that space. Like many of my fellow students, I was most relaxed when I positioned myself at the greatest distance I could get away with—which translated into kicking range or beyond. But my teacher kept a close eye on us. He began requiring us to stay in whatever range we were training, whether it was our favored range or not, making it difficult to stray too far. Our job was to discover our best range(s), but it was equally important to become as skillful as we could in the others and to float between them as the need arose.

Attributes were everything. Those of us who liked to maintain a distance had to cultivate speed and footwork to make ourselves functional. We learned to make ourselves evasive, and to move swiftly. We discovered ways to put everything into a single kick or punch when an opening occurred. Those who liked to be up close had to cultivate more rapid hand movements. They learned to trap an opponent's arms and redirect energy. They had to *resist* putting everything into a single shot and determine how to save some energy for the next.

What is the best range? The answer is manifested in an old martial arts truth that reveals the secret of the great Asian dragon: The dragon is really all of the other martial arts animals combined. The dragon can work both long and short ranges, as well as all the ranges in between. Of course, the lesson is that this is how you and I can also engender the most advantage.

Know your attributes. The more I trained, the more I became aware of my own attributes, especially speed and sensitivity. I began to pay attention to where, in terms of ranges, I could generate the most power; get the better blocks and strikes. As my personal mode of self-expression surfaced, I realized that my comfort and skill zones *were*, in fact, good at a long range, but were even better at close range, which became my first area of specialization. What an irony, considering how, when I began, all I wanted to do was stay as far away from my partners as possible. My original preference for distance training was based on all the wrong reasons. I was running from opponents rather than learning how to work with them. What an exciting eye-opener it was to find that the very space I most feared was the range in which I could shine. This was significant because it made me feel less restricted in both movement and thinking. What a lesson. What a newfound sense of freedom—to feel in control where once I felt controlled.

Experiences such as these are gold mines for building confidence and bringing us closer to our full potentials, whether in martial arts or in everyday life. What is it about life that keeps us looking in the opposite direction from where our true talents await us? The answer is simple: Our fears and other negative emotions play a big role, but mostly we do not give enough voice to our innermost self—to knowing the person we really are on the inside.

In the classroom, it's important for me to identify student ranges—on the first day of class if I can. This makes it easier for me to fine-tune my course in my hope to shape it into a positive experience for as many as possible.

Recognizing students' individual ranges helps me know the space(s) of their greatest potential, as well as their limits. This helps me better get along with them and communicate more. It facilitates getting the best out of them and enables me to avoid many potential problems.

There are always those students who are most comfortable at long ranges. Many times, these students sit in the far recesses of the room. Interestingly, a lot of them know how to make distance work. Long range gives them time to deliberate and plan. When they see an opening they want to fill, they are swift as a crane soaring in to answer questions, or offer opinions and debates.

Then there are those who are comfortable at close range. These students often sit in front. They are eager to get into conversations and debates and don't require as much planning to respond. They don't mind being part of a discussion before they actually have an answer. They are confident that they can create openings and that an answer will come.

Knowing the attributes and limitations of each range helps me customize questions, discussions, and so forth. This way, everyone gets a "target" that he or she can hit. This helps everyone feel good about themselves and fosters a friendly and effective environment.

Further, just as my martial arts instructor did with me, my job is to create activities that provide exploration of other ranges, as well. As each student expands his or her zones for self-expression, the whole group benefits. The overall atmosphere becomes less intimidating, more spontaneous, and more creative.

There are myriads of people living in and through ranges in our everyday routines. Not long ago, a business colleague and I just couldn't connect personally. We became progressively more distant toward each other, although, as life would have it, we still needed to work together for some time. The distance that had grown between us was making business interactions extremely difficult; left unattended, it would eventually render them impossible.

Something had to be done. So I chanced getting closer, a little at a time and delicately. I paid attention to how my colleague talked to others with whom we mutually interacted; to the tone of her words. I discovered that she was not usually emotive, but she *was* personable and conversational, rather than formal. I made myself attentive to how others talked to her and her reactions—when she seemed genuinely excited, when she did not.

I noticed that she liked to be polite, but not personal and certainly not intimate. She liked to float straight down the middle. Interestingly, whenever anyone got too close, she would back off to her most distant range. My close-range skills were misaligned with her mid-range comfort zone.

I decided to wait for an opening to emerge, during which I might try to meet her in her own ranges. In the meantime, I tried to remain present to the attributes of those who had successful relationships with her, and to focus on which of these could most naturally be cultivated in my own rapport.

When the opening occurred, one day during a discussion of business protocol, I seized the moment. I slowly and attentively closed the distance between us by using some of the same language and points of discussion I'd heard others exchanging with her. Being sensitive to her energy, her boundaries and openings, I found that we were able to enjoy a better, healthier, and somewhat *more connected* conversation. Our relationship had eased, even if just to a small extent. Staying on this course, however, I found that our working relationship became considerably less stressed and more trusting. And even though a few occasions arose in which resharpening of these skills was necessary, our overall rapport continued in a positive direction. Our once edgy relationship had become freer and more manageable.

We are all born with a natural aptitude in one or more ranges. Find your range. Expand your comfort zones. Become proficient in as many other ranges as you can. Learn how to float, without hindrance, among them. Keep hold of your center. Like tranquil water, stand attentive between directing yourself and being directed, as if at a point of impartiality—and move from there. You will get the best out of yourself and others.

Meditation
Finding Your Range

*When you look into the eyes of another, any other, and you
see your own soul looking back at you, then you will know
you have reached another level of consciousness.*
                                        —BRIAN WEISS, M.D.

Visualize yourself interacting with various people
within your daily routines. Try to pick one person from
each of the ranges: Choose one who likes to interact
closely, and another who keeps a longer distance. Then
think of two who fit the in-between ranges.

Identify the category in which you feel most comfortable. What attributes do you seem to display in this
range? How do they manifest—in words, tone, mood,
body language, implications of goodwill, or other ways?

Now consider the ranges where you are least comfortable. How does your discomfort manifest? *Note:* You
will know when you're in a space where others are more
proficient because you will feel that they have the upper
hand. If this occurs, observe what attributes they possess
that give them this advantage.

Visualize an assortment of people you encounter in
your daily life. Identify in which of the four ranges they

seem to best operate. Choose one person from each range whom you feel is effective. What attributes enable these individuals to excel?

Consider people with whom each of these aforementioned individuals successfully interrelates. What attributes do they show?

Consider someone in your daily routines with whom you feel you are in conflict. Identify his or her range(s). Then try to visualize yourself using some of the attributes you identified above, in an attempt to get things working more toward your purposes.

Consider someone in your daily routines with whom you feel personable or intimate. Identify his or her range(s). Then try to visualize yourself using some of the attributes you identified above, in an attempt to make things between you even more pleasant.

Know yourself and others and create the right fit for every situation.

Resolutions
Finding Your Range

✧ Today, I will attempt to improve my attributes in all ranges.

✧ Today, I will be present to the various distances I attempt to establish with others and to those they attempt to establish with me.

✧ Today, I will be present to comforts and discomforts (my own and those of others) as I move from one range to another with the people of my life.

✧ Today, I will attempt to identify what attributes others possess when they successfully move from one range to another in their lives.

✧ Today, I will attempt to identify what attributes I possess—and which I require more work on—as I move from one range to another with the people of my life.

✧ Today, I will attempt to enter my ranges for the right reasons.

✧ Today, I will enter the spaces of others softly, attentively, and with respect.

✧ Today, I will attempt to expand my comfort zones.

✧ Today, I will enjoy my freedom and allow others the same.

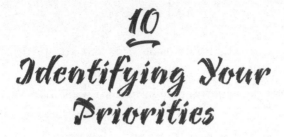

10
Identifying Your Priorities

Consider Your Net Gain

Zen is to have the heart
and soul of a little child.

—TAKUAN

ometimes martial artists become consumed with tagging their opponents in any way they can. The majority of our attention focuses on trying to get in the shot—any shot. We eventually learn, however, that what's important is not necessarily landing a strike, but rather landing an effective one. We soon discover that we may even have to give something up in order to gain some. We learn that not every attack requires a block or even a reaction.

Sometimes what looks great, isn't. False impressions of power won't get you far. Gains, on the mats, are seldom as *theatrical* as what you see in movies. To get the job done, you have to put vanity aside. You have to prioritize and consider the net gains of your actions.

One day while training kicks, I sat watching my teacher work strategies with one of his advanced students. I remember the student launching a low roundhouse—not striking full force, of course—at my instructor's thigh.

"Tactically, what would you do to defend against a kick like that?" the student asked. Everyone wants to know the answers to *What-would-you-do-if* . . . questions. After all, self-defense is one of our primary interests.

"Nothing," the instructor replied.

We all thought that was fairly curious.

"Nothing?" the student pressed him.

"I'd *take* the shot," our instructor said.

I wrongly interpreted his remark as a show of strength; it was rather a show of acceptance.

Once, a high-ranked student was sparring a novice. Every time the senior student executed a combination of kicks, he'd glance over to our instructor, out of the corner of his eye. At one point, the senior student launched a fast, high spinning kick that landed just a few feet short of his opponent. I remember how impressed I was; I'd seen acrobatic kicks like that in films, but never live.

The less experienced student stopped short. "Was that supposed to be an offensive or defensive move?" he asked.

I was confused. Was the less experienced student as unimpressed as he sounded? I looked over to our teacher, who was shaking his head and smiling. "That's just the problem," he answered.

I thought about it and realized that the senior student hadn't really gained anything with his fancy move. Perhaps he had tried to impress the teacher, but even that hadn't worked. His move, which had effected little to no gain, looked impressive only to the untrained eye.

Moreover, the senior student had left himself open to attack because of the shaky positioning afforded by his showy kick—he had lost balance, and there was considerable hesitation before his next move. His "performance" hadn't paid off either on the mats or with our instructor.

One day, my teacher and I were sparring. I wasn't faring very well, to say the least. Whether I stepped in or retreated, his energy flowed with mine. His sensitivity was that powerful. I couldn't flow as well with him, and he was thus able to break rhythm and tag me whenever he felt like it—at least, that was my interpretation of things.

Ironically, to anyone watching, *I* would have appeared the aggressor. And equally as ironic, I was. Why? Because I felt he was in complete control of me even though he wasn't doing much of anything. I, on the other hand, constantly felt that I had to be doing *something* to gain the upper hand. Every time I did—you guessed it—my shot would backfire, and I'd get tagged.

"You have to know the difference between a gain and

a loss," he explained. "It's kind of like playing chess. You're going for the pawns, while I'm going for your queen and king."

It was true. I had to learn to prioritize. The only strikes I ever seemed to take at him were ones I knew could get in, but they were nothing shots and wouldn't net much gain. He could have "taken" them as easily as he could have taken the roundhouse from his other student when I was watching them practice—in fact, I thought, more easily. I knew this because I could have taken them myself.

From that day on, I tried to put vanity aside. Whenever I felt the need to be doing something, anything, to feel I was in control, an alarm sounded in my head, warning me that I had lost sight of my priorities—in which case I was serving myself up on a silver platter.

I went over all the basics *again.* I began to consider real gains, which, as my teacher defined them, were shots that counted.

But you have to look at every circumstance individually. What could be considered a gain in one situation may very well turn out to be a loss in another. As with that notorious roundhouse to the thigh, if the opponent can take the shot, you're not really gaining anything. In fact, you may be playing right into his or her hands. If the opponent *can't* take the shot, however, it may put you in position for a win.

The mats showed me that it was possible to turn losses into gains. Once I realized this, I began testing the concept at every opportunity. For example, instead of becoming anxious for misjudging a move, I worked on staying cool, looking for the real targets, and executing the turnaround—turning the loss to my advantage. I once heard someone say that mistakes were really "Zen blessings."

In many ways, this is true. For instance, you can roll a failed block into an effective punch, turn a botched strike into an unexpected takedown, or miss a kick altogether and launch a surprise leg sweep. As long as you stay alert and don't panic, an error can give you whatever perspective you need to get the job done.

Just get the job done. This popular anthem in martial arts can be applied to life as well. But you have to prioritize and consider net gain. Before you start an action, ask yourself: Is this action necessary to accomplish my goal? Or is it, as the saying goes, an action that could result in your winning the battle and yet losing the war?

One of my household appliances recently went on the blink. When I called the repairman, the first thing he asked was whether the warranty was still good. I didn't know. He suggested that I call the manufacturer. I called their customer-support line during a break in my schedule and was put on hold for the first available technician.

When the technician eventually answered, he abruptly put me on hold and left me there for more than half an hour. At several points during my wait, I was tempted to simply hang up and call another time.

My frustrations deepened. I didn't really think that the warranty would still be in effect, and I began to wonder if I was wasting my time. I was considering saying something to the technician regarding his lack of courtesy when I eventually got through.

That's when I put on the brakes and started going over priorities. I asked myself what I could possibly gain by sustaining my attitude. My goal was to try to get the repair completed under the warranty, no? This was the point of the call, no? I realized that, in the larger scheme of things, waiting was nothing more than "a shot I could easily take." So rather than striking out when the technician returned to the line, I calmed myself and let him speak.

Interestingly, he apologized several times for the long wait. My newly adopted technique was to be as pleasant and attentive as I could. He matched his tone to mine and explained that, unfortunately, my warranty had in fact expired. I kept my composure and said I'd thought that might be the case. In the end, however, he agreed that the problem sounded kind of quirky and so he'd be happy to extend the warranty and cover me for the repair.

Needless to say, I was pleased with the results, especially considering where the situation might have gone.

The solution had come simply and without any real difficulty. Prioritizing and considering net gains had paid off.

Always identify your priorities, whether you are conducting a business transaction, dealing with personal relationships, or considering matters of physical, emotional, and spiritual health. Consider the net gains of your actions. Don't become anxious. Don't move just to move. Stay cool. Look for the real targets. Pick your move. Execute your shot.

Meditation
Identifying Your Priorities

When our actions create discord in another person,
we, ourselves, in this lifetime or another,
will feel that discord.
Likewise, if our actions create harmony
and empowerment in another,
we also come to feel
that harmony and empowerment.

—GARY ZUKAV

Visualize a situation that you feel requires a response from you and that has, despite several attempts, gone on unresolved.

Consider your goal in the aforementioned situation. Then visualize any action steps you are thinking about taking. Ask yourself if such a response is necessary to accomplish your goals. Will the action result in a true gain? Has this action worked with another individual, in a similar situation? Are there differences between these individuals? Between the situations? Why might the action be effective in one case but not be effective in the one under consideration?

Are you going for the pawns or queens and kings?

Visualize how the other person (the person with whom

you are attempting to work things out) is working through the situation. Can you turn any of this individual's actions to your advantage?

Consider where the situation begins to bottleneck or deteriorate. What can you do to keep flowing with the individual? Your objective here is to flow past what's stopping the problem from being resolved and look for resolution downstream.

Visualize yourself able to keep flowing (staying cool, heightening your sensitivity, adjusting and readjusting your ranges and rhythms, all the basics) until you see real opportunity, real gain, and then take it.

Gently absorb the techniques of this meditation into your daily routine.

For further consideration. Visualize situations of warmth and joy in your life. Consider the formula: *Don't become anxious, stay cool, go with the flow, look for the real targets, and execute your shot.* Visualize yourself flowing through such a situation, considering a wider range of actions (targets). Ask yourself if any of these could be more gainful in your attempt to nurture even more warmth and joy from the situation. Visualize yourself flowing into these actions.

Gently absorb the techniques of this meditation into your daily routine.

Resolutions
Identifying Your Priorities

✧ Today, I will try to see my actions and reactions in terms of trade-offs. I will be attentive to the gains and losses presented by each.

✧ Today, I will remember that I do not have to react to every action coming my way.

✧ Today, I will look for opportunities to not react to certain actions in an effort to gain a better position.

✧ Today, I will pay attention to how certain words and actions contribute toward my purposes with specific individuals and not with others. I will attempt to ascertain why.

✧ Today, I will remember that what is effective is not necessarily showy.

✧ Today, I will try to place the full panorama of my life skills behind my decision making.

✧ Today, I will look for opportunities to turn losses into gain. I will try not to become anxious when losing position or intention. I will remain cool, go with the flow, look for real targets, and execute a turnaround whenever possible.

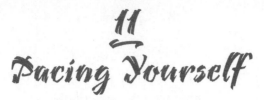

11
Pacing Yourself
Manage Your Energy

*Action is a high road to
self-confidence and self-esteem.*
—BRUCE LEE

*H*aving enough internal energy, *when we
need it*, to do the things we want is
paramount to experiencing life to the
fullest. It seems that everyone, whether on the mats or in
everyday situations, is looking for ways to generate more
energy and methods of conserving it for the long haul. In
martial arts, such energy building and conservation is
accomplished by careful regulation and measurement of
movement, physical and mental—a process known as *pacing*. Good martial artists learn to manage their use of
energy, drawing from it when they need to and simultaneously replenishing their supply.

I remember the first time I tried sparring three rounds
of three minutes apiece. I tired myself out so quickly,

dodging attacks and trying to counter, that in essence I lost the match to my own exhaustion. On the other hand, I couldn't help noticing how most of the senior students looked like they were just warming up after three rounds of the same length. I was amazed. I couldn't figure out where their energy was coming from, or where I was going wrong. I felt deficient—like maybe I couldn't cut it.

One of our routine sparring drills was known as the Dragon's Circle. The purpose of this exercise was to help build endurance and energy management skills. It also familiarized us with a wide variety of opponents and combat styles.

First, our instructor positioned us in a circle. Then he would place one of us in the center. That person (male or female, novice or veteran) would have to spar everyone in the circle, one at a time. Each match lasted until either one or the other student submitted or until the teacher clapped his hands and ended it, sending in the next opponent.

Again, it seemed the novices would tire early and the advanced students would *gain* energy as they went along. I didn't get it.

After class one day, I asked my instructor why I was having such a hard time maintaining stamina. Where was I going wrong? I ran three miles every day, practiced all of my katas and techniques, thought I was in fairly good shape, yet every time I was required to be in the center of the circle, I found myself short on energy—losing many of my matches and exhausting myself even when I won.

"You need to work out the dynamics of your game," he said. "Your *pacing*."

He told me to remember the cardinal rules: *Manage your energy. Move only when necessary and as efficiently as possible, and use only as much force as needed to accomplish your task.*

To develop better management skills, I again went back to basics. By then, I clearly understood that whenever I learned a new martial arts concept, I had to retool all previous ones with every bit of new information, broadening their scope and application. That's the way martial arts work. That's why people choose to make them a permanent part of their lives. They are a never-ending font of nourishment.

It seemed paradoxical—using and storing energy, in essence emptying and filling, in the same moment. I tried cultivating and condensing chi and then using it only when needed. This reduced work strain and seemed a good step forward. But there was still something missing. I wasn't able to generate and store energy while using it at the same time.

It was a good thing I had retooled my basics, because I drew on all of them when my breakthrough came.

Without thinking, I felt my consciousness sinking. I relaxed into a deep state of calmness, though I was about to face my third of twelve opponents. Surprisingly, my attention sharpened. This made sense—too much concentration can cause a loss of attention. All of us have experienced concentrating on one thing so tightly that other people can walk into the room with us and we never even know they are there. Try thinking hard about something and drinking a soda or listening to music. You're bound to miss some of each experience—taste or sound. Once you sink your consciousness, you can see and intuit more.

As for me, it was a though I'd suddenly discovered a second mental hard drive and processor, with many times the memory and speed of the former. I used this *deepened* state of consciousness to direct all my actions, using only the force that was necessary, redirecting wherever possible. I eliminated unnecessary actions whenever feasible, using straight lines and conserving energy to land my targets. Above all, I kept my consciousness downward, summoning and condensing more chi as I went along.

When you are condensing chi, your body works like a transformer and can use the movement itself to create more energy. Thus, I began to condense and recirculate chi to where it was needed in my body, directing breath to my Lower Dan Tien to cultivate more chi, drawing it in from my limbs after each movement, and redistributing it when and where I required.

My whole body felt lighter and more alert. My mind stayed cool, flexibly moving with my opponents' energies.

To my surprise, when the drill was over, I didn't have the *wiped-out-every-muscle-sore-boy-am-I-gonna-be-hurting-tonight* feeling that usually followed an afternoon in the Dragon's Circle. The energy I had cultivated lasted well into the next day.

"When you store energy properly," my teacher said, "you should feel centered and invigorated. Training should leave you feeling powerful enough to redirect a Mack truck coming at you full speed, not like you just got hit by one." I loved that adage, and with more practice, I began to feel what he meant.

I decided to apply these same skills to jogging. I found that, just like on the mats, I could conserve and restore energy while using it. Not only that, but I improved my time and eliminated the usual muscle and joint aches. Further, I was able to retain and use the rich, clean, surplus energy well into the next day.

It didn't take long before I started applying these skills to all types of daily situations, from academic work to business, sports, ordinary chores, and even intimate situations.

Pacing will help you restore and conserve energy as you expend it. Practice whenever and wherever you can.

Meditation
Pacing Yourself

From point comes a line, then a circle;
When the circle is complete,
Then the last is joined to the first.
—SHABISTARI

Consider a recent stressful event, personal or situational. Before you visualize the details:

✧ Center.

✧ Relax and regulate your breathing.

✧ Feed your mind positive energy, creating a mental image that empowers you. Use a totem of your choice—tiger, leopard, crane, or the like; or you may want to use a character from a movie. Either way, what you're striving for is the feeling of invincible strength delivered through your totem, which you can absorb.

Now begin to play the stressful event in your mind like a movie. Imagine yourself moving through the situation and dealing with it calmly and naturally.

✧ Sink your energy. Let your sensitivity heighten and remain cool.

✧ Analyze the situation, gathering and conserving chi. Keep your purpose clear in your mind.

✧ Then respond with an economy of motion and efficient use of energy when the appropriate openings occur.

✧ Gather and recirculate chi when and where necessary.

Recycle these steps until you have reached a positive outcome.

Alternate version. Use the aforementioned meditation, except imagine a positive situation instead of a stressful one. See how following the suggested pattern for pacing can heighten an already positive experience.

Gently practice these skills throughout the day on the various individuals you encounter. See how you can freely move in and out of conversation and better direct it toward your goals.

Resolutions
Pacing Yourself

✧ Today, I will remember to relax periodically and feed myself positive energy throughout my daily routines.

✧ Today, I will remember that if I try to "muscle" things, I will only tire.

✧ Today, I will remember that energy is saved by using my skills.

✧ Today, I will try to expend energy only when it leads to positive results.

✧ Today, I will attempt to accomplish my goals in as few motions as possible.

✧ Today, I will appropriate only what energy is necessary to accomplish my goals.

✧ Today, I will attempt to eliminate as much hesitation from my mental and physical movements as possible.

✧ Today, I will remember that it is all right to change my plans in order to move more naturally and fluidly with the problems and joys that will arise.

✧ Today, I will gather and conserve energy as I flow through the events of my life.

✧ Today, I will remain centered in my joys as well as my difficulties. I will follow my center, which always directs me—like a compass—to my bliss and to the Infinite.

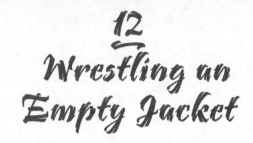

12
Wrestling an Empty Jacket

Overcome Force with Softness

When a man is living,
he is soft and supple.
When he is dead,
he becomes hard and rigid.

—TAO TE CHING

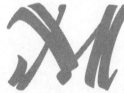any martial arts techniques are inspired by nature. For example, a force the size of a tornado can snap telephone poles and pulverize houses, yet a blade of grass or a leaf can make surviving such rage look effortless and graceful. Every martial arts student will eventually hear one version of this story or another, several times over. Why? Because it is so important, yet so easily forgotten. What is soft and flexible can withstand great force. What is brittle, breaks.

In the martial arts, the words *hard* and *soft* are traditional terms used to distinguish between two distinct styles and philosophies.

- ✧ Internal or soft styles (such as Tai Chi, Judo, and Aikido) focus on the development of mind and spirit, or *internal* strength and energy (chi), as well as the redirection of force rather than meeting it head-on.

- ✧ External or hard styles (Tae Kwon Do and Karate) focus on *external* conditioning of muscular strength, body movement, and the application of external force.

It must be said that most martial arts contain elements of each, and a good martial artist will know how to employ softness and stillness as well as force. Still, the ability to overcome force (such as a tornado's) with minimum effort (as a blade of grass or a leaf) is the focal point of *internal* or *soft* systems of martial arts.

There is a legendary story about how an opponent of the great Judo player Jigoro Kano (founder of Judo) once described competing against Kano as *trying to fight an empty jacket.* The comparison perfectly expresses the nature and effect of softness as a martial arts technique. Simply put, you overcome force with softness.

If your experience is anything like mine, then you know that a major concern among individuals, families, institutions—the entire nation, really—is the amount of stress we are hit with every day, from all directions. It's easy to say, "Loosen up," but the tensions of contemporary life can drive us far from what it means to be truly soft. Sometimes it's difficult to remember what real softness is. But every now and then, something happens that shows us just how rigid we've become. That's a good time to pay attention; to see how far we've drifted from our natural state of softness, the one we were born into. That is the time to take measurement and to reprogram our actions.

I remember the first time I was Judo-thrown. A woman half my size flung me to the mats as if I was no challenge at all. I fell like a bag of rocks, my hip and elbows crashing to the ground. The instructor noticed.

"You keep falling like that, and you're going to get hurt," he said.

"Going to?" I chuckled, massaging my elbow.

He laughed. "You're all resistance. You have to soften up."

I wasn't exactly sure what he meant by *soften.* When I executed the same throw on my partner, however, I noticed that from contact to takedown, she became loose as silk, offering no resistance whatsoever. Her body seemed so weightless she might as well have been invisible. All I could feel was the smooth energy of its motion, as if she had attached herself to movement, as if she had *become* the movement. I remembered Jigoro Kano's story. There it was, I thought, the notorious empty jacket, weightless as a leaf.

If you want to overcome force, get soft. Silky light, my partner was able to simply accept the throw, maintaining balance and actually gaining advantage in her positioning, had she wanted to counter my move.

Again, I found myself learning a lesson about control. Even though I had initiated the action, she apparently was the one in charge. I was beginning to see that softness had a deeper level. I realized (in terms of application) that the mythic jacket may be empty, but nonetheless it is sensitive and conscious. Still, I remained puzzled.

She told me it was all about getting loose, really loose, void yet fully attentive. "You have to practice not being afraid to take the throw," she said. "If you have any apprehensions, you'll never get loose enough. The fall," she continued, "is part of the movement. It's where you and the movement become one."

In time and with plenty of practice, I began to gain more confidence in *falling*. I stopped resisting being thrown and allowed myself to become weightless in the movement. This strategy would almost always reposition me in a place of advantage. But I learned that we have to stay soft and wait for the repositioning, and it has to occur naturally. And as long as we stay nonresistant and harmonize with the motion, we avoid the full shock of impact. Eventually, we reduce the odds of getting hurt, and with that, reduce our anxieties. That, of course, opens a whole new door to gaining advantageous positions as we work toward our goals.

Once we realize the power of weightlessness, we'll want to incorporate it into everything we do. I began training in weightlessness. I started by imagining my limbs loose as spaghetti. But my instructor cautioned, "Don't think of softness as limp or weak; you'll get into trouble that way. The softness we're talking about is intensely alert on the surface, yet underneath it is strong as steel."

I, like many people, had forgotten what true softness felt like. When I told him the paradox confused me, he suggested that I practice my katas in a lake or pool to better understand.

"Once you experience what I'm talking about," he said, "remember the feeling. Then transfer it into practice."

A couple of weeks later, I was vacationing in the Adirondacks and decided to head for one of the Lake George beaches. There were a lot of people at the beach that day, but I couldn't help myself; I just had to see what my teacher was talking about when he mentioned doing katas in water. I felt a little foolish, but I figured a few inconspicuous arm movements wouldn't attract any attention. So I found myself a spot that was out of view, and gave it a whirl.

The experience gave me what I was missing in my workouts. My arms floated weightlessly and soft as sleeves gliding on the water. They were alert and light, yet I could feel (as my teacher had described) their steely power, calm and attentive inside them. Light as they were, they still felt strong. The softer and lighter they felt externally, the harder and stronger they felt internally. You can literally feel your bones strengthening. When you are full of tension, the feeling is just the opposite.

The concepts I had been studying were starting to come together. I was beginning to understand: Chi fuels *floating power* into action, breath directs chi, and the sunken mind is what directs your breath.

The concept of *empty jacket* has both liberated and empowered me in life many times. Practice it, and you will not intimidate. You cannot be sucked into disputes. You will be free to be completely who you are, even when the forces around you are trying to storm you elsewhere. Just remember: If you want to overcome force, get soft.

It was morning rush hour, and I was stranded in a median, along with two other cars, waiting to pull into a gas station. The young woman ahead of me was having trouble shooting into traffic, and it soon became obvious that she was learning how to drive. When she remained in the median for a while longer than what was comfortable, the young man she was with motioned me and the driver behind me to go aound them. But just then, their car jerked forward and stalled.

Then the fellow behind me belligerently laid on his horn, and the guy in front stuck his head out the car window and yelled obscenities in my direction. He had concluded that I was the one who'd honked at him.

As luck would have it, I wound up behind him in line waiting to pay for gas. He shifted his weight from side to side and seemed ironically impatient as he waited for the cashier. I fervently hoped that he wouldn't notice me. I tried to relax. It's amazing how loose you can get just by thinking yourself there. But he did turn and notice me, and unleashed a fit of foul language. He had become inflexible and bristly. So what could I do? I chose to glide with his words as though I were weightless as Kano's empty jacket. I gave him nothing to argue with. What he thought of me was insignificant. I rolled with all he threw at me and didn't let any of the impact penetrate.

Eventually he emptied himself of hostilities. In the end, he'd gotten no reaction out of me, and when he looked to the cashier for agreement, the cashier simply feigned a smile. No reaction there, either. Neither of us had been receptive to the hostile man's fit. He had intimidated no one. When he was done wielding his anger like a knife with nothing to cut into, he simply left. He had defeated himself.

Conflict is never fun to deal with, but you can roll with the movement. Trust in the process. Respond to force with softness. The perpetrator will eventually tire and extinguish or will leave you at a place of advantage, from which you can accomplish your goals.

Meditation
Wrestling an Empty Jacket

Heaven and earth do nothing,
yet there is nothing
which they do not accomplish.
—CHUANG-TSE

Place yourself in water—a tub, pool, lake, or the like. Breathe gently and relax. Let your arms float horizontally. Then begin to move them back and forth and feel their weightlessness. Feel the steely strength inside them. Keep moving them. Concentrate on your Lower Dan Tien. On your out-breath, direct your chi into your arms as you move them back and forth.

Now direct your chi to your fingertips and hold it there for a moment; then, in concentrations spatially no bigger than a quarter, to your palms; then to your wrists; to a spot midway between your wrists and your elbows; and finally to your elbows. *Try visualizing the directed chi as a dot similar to a point of sunlight filtered through a magnifying glass.*

Repeat this exercise as many times as you like. Try it with your eyes closed.

Note how you can concentrate chi anywhere on your body. Further, note your body's suppleness. This is the softness you want to strive for during everyday conflicts. Allow your mind the same suppleness.

Additional version. Visualize someone with whom you are or have been in conflict. Soften yourself physically and mentally—become like an empty jacket riding each wave of conflict cast by that individual; become one with the movement until the person tires and extinguishes or the movement itself gives you the upper hand. Watch as the person grows frustrated, unable to bully you, and eventually defeats him- or herself.

Resolutions
Wrestling an Empty Jacket

✧ Today, I will remember that the tiniest of leaves can endure the most powerful of winds by becoming part of the movement rather than fighting it.

✧ Today, I will avoid fueling the hostilities of others. Instead I will practice falling into their movements until they extinguish or place me in a position of advantage.

✧ Today, I will remember that even spiritual and emotional falls can be harmonized to land us in better positions.

✧ Today, although it may be difficult, I will attempt to soften myself periodically—body, mind, and spirit. I will enjoy the ease and grace of my actions.

✧ Today, I will remember that to be one with each moment, one with each movement, I must stay empty. I will remember the paradox—that in my emptiness, I will experience the fullness and presence of all things.

✧ Today, I will remember that softness is the state I was born into and the most natural state in which to live.

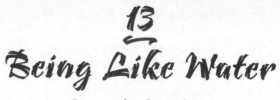

13
Being Like Water
Go with the Flow

If nothing within you stays rigid,
outward things will disclose themselves.
Moving, be like water. Still, be like a mirror.
Respond like an echo.

—BRUCE LEE

Going with the flow is the martial artist's way. The experienced martial artist doesn't think in terms of *means-to-an-end*. Instead, he or she begins to live wholly in the present, participating in each moment as it comes, moving with what *is*. *Way* and *end* become the same movement, and that is: to harmonize. All learned forms and techniques become one living movement able to adapt to any situation.

To go with the flow, learned form evolves into free form, and you become spontaneous. The martial artist has reached the level of expert.

To go with the flow, rather than to interfere with action, you become part of it, allowing things to take their natural course. You are like the mirror surface of undisturbed water—your mind still and awake, reflecting everything, lovely or dreadful, without allowing any of it to spoil the calm. This mind-set is known as *mizu no kokoro* or "mind like water."

To go with the flow, you become tranquil and peaceful. You strive to always and everywhere *be like water*—for water can be all things: gentle and powerful, still and in motion, floating and floated upon, heavy, light, invisible, solid, and vapor.

To go with the flow, people appear carefree as they float from one range to another, their actions relaxed, serene. Water people are soft on the outside and strong on the inside.

To go with the flow, you must slay the ego. Joseph Campbell, in *The Power of Myth*, defined *ego* as "what you think you want, what you will to believe, what you think you can afford, what you decide to love, what you regard yourself bound to." He went on, "It may all be too small, in which case it will nail you down. . . . Ultimately, the last deed [slaying the ego] has to be done by you." The greatest combat martial artists (and all aspiring water people) must face is with themselves.

The way to slay the ego is to sink your consciousness and do everything from there—everything. The centered mind is balanced, stable, and egoless. It is connected to everything and everyone because it flows from the

Infinite, the foundation of all energy, the source of all consciousness.

The water mind is liberated and at peace. It is aware and quick and intelligent. It is boundless, and thus, you cannot be *nailed down* as long as you can maintain it.

Water people are soft, egoless, natural, and ever-changing.

Several years after I had begun my studies in martial arts, some time after water had become my guiding metaphor, my instructor had asked me to work out with him one on one. I remember that it was a beautiful, hot midsummer afternoon. We had decided to go outside and practice chi sao.

I had been trying to maintain high doses of positive energy and to live life as softly as possible. My sensitivity was good. I felt strong and healthy—physically and spiritually.

I suppose you could say that life and art were both good that day and, perhaps, quite merged. My teacher and I were smoothly moving through our drill. We had practiced this exercise for years, and I had never, even once, gotten a shot in on him—well, not one that would *count.* "When you land one of those shots," he once explained, "you and your opponent both know it."

So there we were moving along, taking shots, redirecting, flowing together. I didn't feel the usual tension of momentarily losing control, which I often felt when he and I practiced chi sao. I didn't feel I had to be doing anything in particular, either—just staying in the flow seemed right. The longer we repeated the movement, the more I could sense our energy heightening. Then suddenly harmony broke. The next thing I felt was the thrust of a forward shot my teacher had launched, and like water coolly cascading over rock, I—without any thought whatsoever—rolled my forearm over the top of it and countered with a smooth, high strike that landed perfectly on target.

Form had evolved into free form. I'd tagged him.

For a moment, everything seemed in slow motion. I couldn't believe what had occurred. There it was, I thought, the shot that I'd been looking for. He had always said that one day this would happen and how, when it did, it would honor both his teaching and my learning.

Neither of us said a thing. But then I saw the sudden burst of delight in his face as he freely and cordially acknowledged my strike as an excellent one. He congratulated me with much sincerity and went on to tell me just how far I had come along.

I realized yet another lesson was at hand. In going with the flow, we should acknowledge successes in life, whether they are our own or someone else's; by accepting them, we participate with them, becoming part of them in harmony; and then we move on, softly, egolessly, and naturally—like water, fluid and ever-flowing.

What I didn't know was that there was another celebration yet to come. But for that, I was going to have to
wait.

Off the mats, I have made the axiom "be like water"
my guiding light in all that I do. Whether it is attempting
to complete a demanding job, dealing with difficult relationships or personal struggles, or trying to heighten an
already joyful situation, remembering to be like water has
made my life easier and happier.

I remember in particular one difficult interpersonal
relationship that involved a community group whose
members had recently split over a strong political agenda.
Half the group wanted to remove one of the organiza-
tion's leading members and the other half attempted to
sustain his position. I was brand new to the community,
as well as the group. Of course, each faction was working
hard to drag me to its side of the fight.

My objectives, however, were different from either
alliance's. As a result, each time I felt someone trying to
pull me to his or her side of the issue, I became supple,
flowing around the manipulation and gently voicing my
opinions when an opening appeared.

A great attribute of water is that it can transform to
fit into any environment and situation and still remain
entirely itself. I trusted in the tenets of water to get me to
where I needed to be. There were times in my community
group when I had to become nearly invisible in order to

avoid being pinned down by the animosity that was spreading beyond the person who was the focus of their separation—and now to each other. During harsher moments, I remained as fluid as possible so that I could flow around talk that had hardened, and whenever I could, redirect it with softer, lighter conversation. Other times, it was best to be still and reflecting, neither allowing anything to stick nor absorbing anything personally. Eventually, the controversial member resigned of his own volition, and I learned that I didn't have to cave in to other people's manipulation. I could be a free thinker, maintaining an objective and clear mind, and still fully participate with those around me.

One of my favorite examples of going with the flow is tracing the events that have led me to places of satisfaction. I urge you to do this with anything that has brought you joy and happiness. If your experience has been like mine, once you begin to connect the dots, you will see how so many of the difficult situations and people that have drifted in and out of your life, in the end, have been an integral part of what has brought you happiness. One particular example comes to mind, of a friend who left her employment without another job on the horizon. She was unsure of what awaited around the bend, yet trusted that life would carry her to where she needed to be. She remained relaxed and centered as she flowed from one job possibility to the next. Shortly thereafter, she found new employment that has resulted in a stimulating and nurturing career.

Trust in this process. It may be difficult at first, but the more we make ourselves aware of such movement in our lives, the more gracefully and fearlessly we will learn to live.

In life, just like on the mats, there are bound to be plenty of setbacks as well as successes. Practice going with the flow, and you will attain the greatest levels of cooperation and purpose in each. Be present, be confident, be spontaneous, and be free.

Above all, be like water.

Meditation
Being Like Water

Nothing in the world is softer
and weaker
than water;
But for attacking the hard and strong,
there is nothing like it!
For nothing can take its place.

—LAO-TZU

Think of as many characteristics of water as you can, and then list them in a notebook or journal. Now pick one and imagine implementing it (using *all* the martial arts concepts we have discussed in this book so far) toward one situation of conflict, as well as one situation of joy, in order to better the outcomes of each.

Try employing this property of water into your daily routines. See what happens.

Then go on to the next characteristic, and so on.

Resolutions
Being Like Water

✧ Today, I will try to keep my body and spirit as formless as water. I will attempt to take the shape of whatever spaces I enter.

✧ Today, I will try, whenever I can, to take the path of least resistance.

✧ Today, I will move my consciousness downward and try to do as much as possible from that vantage point.

✧ Today, I will try not to muscle anything.

✧ Today, I will try to remember that harmony means yielding to force.

✧ Today, I will try to let go of all I have learned and trust that it will flow out of me naturally when the need arises.

✧ Today, I will try to keep my mind as still as a smooth lake, reflecting everything that comes to it, letting all float over its surface.

✧ Today, I will remember that only I can decide what's right or wrong for me; no one else can.

✧ Today, I will remember that concepts must be transferred into living movement or else they are just defunct ideas.

✧ Today, I will remember that in yielding to a force outside myself, I am in harmony with the Infinite.

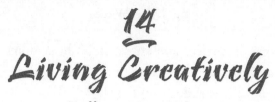

14
Living Creatively
Follow Your Bliss

That which is Bliss is truly the Self.
Bliss and the Self are not distinct
and separate
but are one and identical.
And That alone is real.

—Sri Ramana Maharshi

reative living is approaching life awakened and conscious of who we are, as well as maintaining a deep respect and compassion for others. It is living completely in the moment, happy and free. It is an alternative to the endless cycle of waking up every day in dread of what we must face, reluctantly going through the motions of our routine, then going home at the day's end and finding a way to numb ourselves asleep. Creative living is about getting up each morning excited over the choices that will open to us and the many unexpected places we will go. It is about gathering strength to float through the lulls and energy to make the highs even more enjoyable. It is about minimizing durations of anxiety and stress. It is about doing good work and staying in balance. It is about changing ourselves and the world.

As we begin to live creatively, we return to our primal state of peace and tranquility and follow our bliss. We begin to express ourselves more naturally, initiating change in our lives and in those of the people around us. We are truthful. We become optimistic and direct and thankful. We live simply, in accordance with our true nature. Our job becomes the art of fitting in with all that we are. We seek to feel part of all things and to see the Infinite in them.

The martial arts provide us with self-empowering philosophical skills that can set us unconditionally free to reach our fullest potential, and live our lives as creatively as possible. Traditionally, our various steps of achievement are marked with different colored belts that range from white to black.

Each phase of *Be Like Water* has been intended to accompany you on this journey. I encourage you to mark your level of achievement in terms of belt color as you progress toward your own black belt in life:

❖ White belt: You want more out of life and seek to achieve it.

❖ Yellow belt: You discover that there are techniques that are useful in attaining what you wish to achieve.

✧ Orange belt: You learn these techniques one at a time.

✧ Purple belt: You begin to apply these techniques with the expectation of achieving what you are after.

✧ Blue belt: You see that all techniques merge together as you participate from one moment of living to the next.

✧ Green belt: You realize that these techniques are intended to create harmony with all of life, not to overpower or hurt it.

✧ Brown belt: You stop thinking in terms of technique and simply go after what you need to get done in life without disrupting the natural order of things.

✧ Black belt: You learn to do not only without doing, but without expectation as well.

As we reach the advanced stages of our art, we learn that martial arts are more about living than they ever were about fighting—they're a complete system of mythologies or life lessons that, when applied, can help us become whole and get the most from our lives.

Once we realize this, our quest shifts and becomes a journey toward the bliss and rapture of life, to more fully experience how magnificent it is to be a living creature among other living beings—not just talk about it.

We begin to use our philosophy to become strong internally, rinsing conflict and anxiety from our lives whenever we can. We quest for wholeness, allowing our strengthened spirit to become visible in our daily lives. We become less afraid of rejection and more in favor of expressing who we really are, allowing others the same empowerment.

We realize the point of all our training has been to prepare us to defeat those forces that have restricted us. We understand that the greatest combat we will ever face—that for which we have trained for from the beginning—is against that force *in us* that has kept us from being everything we are and can be. And so we will use the full measure of what we have learned to "slay the dragon of our ego."

Egoless, we realize that our true consciousness, which we refer to as our higher consciousness, is unimaginably vast and quick. Once awake, we cannot go back to sleep. Here we know our innermost self. We *are* our innermost self.

Now, fully conscious of who we are, we open to endless creative possibilities of one living moment to the next. Our focus shifts to the *art* in *martial arts.* Thus begins the martial artist's passage into *creative living,* into the celebration of the beauty of who we truly are within the context of all life.

Art becomes life—completely receptive and expressive. Life becomes art.

Whatever you do, participate. Follow your bliss.

Feeling alive and creating your own choices is what's important. Just keep participating.

Throughout the years, many martial arts colleagues have told me that if it wasn't for the philosophies we trained in, they wouldn't have survived the obstacles life doled out to them—things like loss of employment, hospice care for family members, separation, all kinds of disagreements, and so on. But I hear many tales of heightened joy, as well: stories of relationships, health, and all levels of personal growth.

The fulcrum of these everyday triumphs is in our ability to harmonize our inner and outer life and in making a kindred spirit of the Infinite. When we flow from here, we participate, we are most natural, we nourish and receive nourishment. Strength and healing will come without our seeking.

Just keep following your bliss. For me, as I began to shift my focus from combat to aesthetics, I began to use the movements of my art as meditations—lightening my spirit beyond all prospect. My instructor once told me that this stage of interest is typical of the many who explore their martial art beyond the purpose of self-defense.

"One day you realize your goal is to make beauty of your art," he said.

I took immense pleasure in this phase of training. I felt as if I were no longer simply playing the instrument of my art, but rather using it to compose something for

which I'd been looking for some time: beauty. I was starting to understand: Out of harmony comes beauty, and
out of beauty comes harmony.

Then the major epiphany: I could experience this
feeling of beauty and conscious connectiveness within *any*
of life's movements. I could compose beauty simply by
walking down the street or talking on the phone or cutting wood and stacking logs or jogging or doing anything.
I realized that all of life's movements are our *form,* our *kata*
(and perhaps the highest level of kata).

Follow your bliss. Choose to live consciously and
from the center. Let the excitement of being alive come
pouring out of you. Flow in and through every moment,
creating the masterpiece of your life.

Follow your bliss. Sink so deeply into your center that
you experience a consciousness devoid of thought—an
intuition that is illuminated with awareness. This is who
you are at your deepest. Let *this* consciousness guide you;
allow yourself to grow and change with it. As long as you
can move from there, you will know your bliss. Let it
enlighten you.

Once you've found your bliss, don't lose contact. Create a
sacred space where you can go every day, even for a short
time—half an hour or so. Use your sensitivity to listen to
your Self and trust what comes out of that. Bring this
experience back into your everyday life. Flow from there.

Follow that. See how you begin to live forever changed, more spontaneously, more excitedly connected to everything and everyone in your environment.

Beyond this, we must take care of ourselves in gratitude for our gift of life and consciousness. We make the world a better place by beginning with ourselves, agreeing to experience and absorb as much of life as we can and allowing that to effect change and growth in us. One of the greatest gifts we can return to the world is the fully developed voice of our unique awareness.

Do good deeds. Float goodness toward yourself and back out to others. Think positive and fill the spaces you enter with good energy.

Be well, no matter what. When you are most blissful, you'll want to do good simply for its own beauty. People are drawn to positive energy—and so is cooperation. When you are most centered, you will share positive energy without expectation.

Bliss can't help but flow from a place of balance. If you seek balance, follow your bliss.

Don't be afraid of change. People change, and so does their energy. Creative living is learning to make art of life's changes.

Whether in life or on the mats, the key to dealing with change is to avoid collision of similar energies.

Here is an example: It is better to harmonize yang (hardness, fullness, action, productivity) with yin (softness, emptiness, nonaction, reproductivity) and redirect. Allowed to take their natural course, each opposite force will eventually become the other. Soft will become hard; hard, soft. Action will rest; rest will turn into action. Knowing will become not knowing. Not knowing will become knowing. This is the cycle of life.

Just follow your bliss. Bliss is primal; it is natural. It is you.

Participate and live creatively. Be your Self. Remember, good energy is contagious. Gravitate toward it. Do good. Make beauty. Keep flowing. Follow your bliss.

Meditation
Living Creatively

The earth is my Mother.
The Sky is my Father.
I am a child
of Universal Love.
              —Barbara DeAngelis

Center yourself and let your consciousness sink downward. Visualize yourself speaking to someone you feel comfortable with. Consider qualities about this person that make you feel good and allow the conversation to naturally gravitate there. Stay centered. When an opportunity arises to commend these qualities, do so. Let this arise from your most inward self. Still centered, allow something of yourself that does not surface every day, yet feels intuitively right for this situation, into your rapport. See what new places this takes your relationship.

Try employing this principle in your daily routines. Be receptive to the possibilities.

Alternate version. Create a sacred space in your home, somewhere you can go undisturbed for fifteen to thirty minutes a day. It doesn't have to be anything fancy. The idea is to make a place that offers you quiet and privacy. If you want, put on some favorite music or light a candle or incense or put up some artwork—as long as it makes you feel good, go ahead. If such a space doesn't exist, try someplace outside your home, either out of doors or inside, that's welcoming and comfortable. The point here is to get yourself away from all those things that want something from you during the day and allow yourself to shut the door on them for a while.

Enter this space and be present with yourself. It may take a few minutes to quiet your thoughts and get centered. Trust the process. Let any ideas float through your mind without judgment. Sink your consciousness and simply wait. See what comes forth. Allow yourself to believe what you need is coming to you at this moment.

Notice the relationship between what you discover and what others want from you. They may or may not be the same. Use this information to help you make better choices when opportunities arise.

Another version. Consider someone with whom you are in conflict. Decide whether the energy he or she is putting out is yin or yang. Visualize yourself harmonizing with that person by meeting this energy with the appropriate dynamic of its opposite. But remember, the key is to stay in harmony, not to disrupt.

Then imagine giving that person all the time needed to play out his or her energy.

Now visualize meeting it with the appropriate dynamic of its new opposite.

If necessary, visualize yourself entering and attempting to effect change. Or, if things have already become favorable, visualize yourself maintaining the new flow of energy as it comes into fruition.

Resolutions
Living Creatively

✧ Today, I will create a sacred space and spend time there centering myself.

✧ Today, I will be sensitive to the potential transformation of all things, remembering that my life, too, is open to change and possibility.

✧ Today, I will sink my consciousness and try to do as much as possible from that vantage point.

✧ Today, I will approach my life awakened and conscious of who I am.

✧ Today, I will try to allow others the space and support they need to resolve their own problems.

✧ Today, I will try to approach all my daily encounters confidently and optimistically.

✧ Today, I will recognize the importance of options when responding to conflict.

✧ Today, I will try to do good without anticipation of any reward.

✧ Today, I will try to harmonize the appropriate energy at the right time.

✧ Today, I will honor my connection to all things.

✧ Today, I will honor the Infinite in all things.

✧ Today, I will honor the Infinite in myself.

15
Cultivating Spirituality
Seek Enlightenment

*When the soul strips off
its created nature,
there flashes out
its uncreated prototype.*

—MEISTER ECKHART

he wonderful spiritual teacher and psychologist Ram Dass writes of the paradox of being human, "We are not human beings having a spiritual experience. We are spiritual beings having a human experience." We live in a society that is so fast paced and changing that it often affords little attention to nurturing the spirit. Yet it is the nourishing and freeing of spirit that will lead to our true power as individuals (as well as a people) and bring us happiness and connection to all things.

One of the greatest gifts of the martial arts is that they ultimately guide us to new levels of spirituality. Everything we learn leads to this destination—for the supreme purpose of martial arts ever since Bodhidharma introduced them to the Shaolin monks nearly two centuries years ago has been: *Seek enlightenment.*

But what is enlightenment?

The idea of enlightenment is ever-present in your training. So it's normal to wonder about what it may be and when the day will arrive when you finally experience it. It's not one of those things you can go looking for, like a lost set of car keys. Thus, you must do all the right things, trust in the process, and simply keep flowing.

Then one day, something happens: You feel a jolt in your very center and you realize that it has come from something outside of you. You discover that here is a power that has been with you since birth, and it can facilitate everything you do, and it has surfaced.

Many years ago, my instructor was trying to get me to understand that just as you can hold your hands before your Lower Dan Tien and feel chi between them, you can also move your hands a few inches above any of your limbs and feel chi pouring forth.

"It is only more apparent in the Lower Dan Tien," he explained, "because that is the major location of chi in the body. Actually," he added, "you can move your hands in this way and feel chi radiating from everything around you."

As with many of his ideas, he had thrown out the net

to see if it was going to pull me in. If it did, we would talk about it later, once I'd had a chance to mull it over.

Then, when I least expected, it happened: I was practicing a speed drill on my wooden dummy. (This traditional Kung Fu apparatus has three arms—two upper, one middle—and a leg; it's used for toe-to-toe combat techniques.) I remember working the drill much longer than usual. My arms were exhausted and taking a pounding. It really didn't seem that I could go on much more.

I entered a state of intense mental stillness. My consciousness sank, *naturally.* My breathing, rather than revving, slowed down. Reflexively and from my center, I felt my chi circulate to my limbs, especially my arms. I was suddenly not tired at all. Instead, I was able to torque the drill without effort. It was as though I could feel the oak arms of the apparatus with my aura; as though my own arms were made of conscious light. What's more, I felt my energy being fueled by energy beyond myself, as though I'd tapped into (and drawn from) a source of power capable of nourishing me, as well as protecting me from injury. At first, it all felt automatic, but then I realized I could direct this energy simply by willing it, using all my martial skills to pull it from below me and above me (heavens and earth) at once.

The experience was powerful and vital. Feeling something real and undeniable like that will drive you deeper into your quest for spiritual explorations. This is the way of martial arts. Such experiences will make you hungry for more, fast. That day, my experience—my first—was awesome to me. I'd felt a power beyond that of bone, muscle, or chemistry fueling me, and once you feel a thing like that, you don't forget it. You become curious as to what else can be done with it.

Everyone's breakthrough experience is different. The point, however, is to be patient and to remain receptive. Your job is to practice and trust in your skills and to invite such an experience into your life. It will come. And when it does, you will know it immediately.

Once you begin to experience spirit, don't forget how you got there. For me, the next time I worked out, I had to find a way to get back. This time I tried another route— my forms. What I found was that the movements and postures increased my chi, as well as its flow.

Further, I discovered I could extend my chi a few inches beyond my body. This wasn't something I had to think about; I just started doing it as though it was the most natural thing in the world. It was as involuntary and unpremeditated as a heartbeat. Since then, I've come to realize that there is intelligible energy inside each of us, and its instinctive destination is to flow beyond us.

The feeling of extending chi is somewhat describable. It begins with projecting your consciousness forward, from the Lower Dan Tien. From there, you flow into a space of nothingness, yet, at the same time, somethingness that is completely alert. It is a state of total comfort.

It is tempting to envision this as the movement of an electrical sphere, especially since so many words used to describe these experiences are linked to the movement of electricity: *current, flow, connection, ground,* and more. But this would only limit the experience and our understanding of it. Whenever we experience spirit, we have already transcended words, but not our ability to comprehend. Who among us can say all that a kitten's purr communicates? Words cannot do justice to the experience. Yet our body knows exactly what it means. And so it is with chi. Although our sunken consciousness, which needs no words, can comprehend it entirely.

Several months after I began experimenting with extending chi, I again questioned my instructor about spirituality. I felt that I was entering an area of martial arts most practitioners simply didn't talk about—at least few in my circle of friends did. I wasn't sure how he was going to react. But he told me that he was glad to hear that my skills had carried me to this stage of interest.

He told me, "This is the beginning of what martial arts is finally all about."

He encouraged me to continue using form as a transit into spirit. In fact, he told me to visualize each form I practiced as if it were the only movement in the universe.

"Try to see every posture as a celebration. Go wher-ever that takes you," he said.

He explained the seven chakra points (psychological centers) located along the spine:

1. At the rectum: drives our instinct to survive.

2. In the pelvic area: drives our urge to procreate.

3. Behind the solar plexus: drives our will and urge to conquer, master, or achieve.

4. In the center of the chest: drives emotional healing, compassion, and love.

5. In the throat: drives communication.

6. In the center of the forehead: drives perception.

7. At the crown of the head: drives the spirit.

He encouraged me to take a mental inventory of my needs and to use our regulated breathing techniques to stimulate (massage) the chakra centers that drive those areas. For instance, if I needed more aggression, I could use my breath to favor the chakra center behind the solar plexus.

"On another level," he explained, "you can use chakra points to project energy, sending it outward, and receive energy from any source outside yourself."

I have learned that certain situations have a way of automatically amplifying our capabilities of extending chi, and we can learn from them. On the mats this often occurs in the heat of combat, when your mind is so alert you've already seen, blocked, and countered an opponent's moves before he or she has even done anything and is still standing five feet away from you. You make all the right moves automatically before your opponent has a chance to complete his or hers.

Similar actions occur in everyday life. Have you ever thought of someone intensely, especially when the underlying reason is emotional, and then heard from that person shortly thereafter—say, in a letter or phone call? The usual reply is something like, "Oh, I was just thinking of you." Or, "I've been thinking a lot about you lately." Have you ever stared at someone and had the person turn around as if he or she had felt your gaze? He or she probably *did* feel you or, more precisely, your chi.

Like my encounter with the wooden dummy, if you start mapping what you experience in mind, body, and spirit when these sensations occur, you will learn how to duplicate the movement of energy within you at will or, better yet, make it automatic. This, of course, is what fires our ability to extend and receive chi into whatever areas of our lives we wish.

There are, as well, other things that can be done to facilitate this process of extending and receiving chi:

> ✧ Sinking is essential to this function. Controlling your lungs—making yourself hypersensitive to the air in them as you breathe—helps tighten

your focus and will enable you to sink more smoothly.

✧ If you can create an anchor, you will be able to sink even quicker: anything from holding your hand to your Lower Dan Tien (or wherever you wish to direct your breath) to imagining a small sphere of light moving within your body, tapping the location with your fingertips. Or as Fred L. Miller, author of *How to Calm Down*, says, just "Take the elevator down."

✧ From there, you can use your breath to stimulate any of your chakras, using them to send an abundance of energy to their respective areas of the body. Locations are chosen according to need.

✧ Further, we have the ability to move, project, receive, and share specific energies and consciousness from any or all of our chakras, as well as from the Lower Dan Tien. Consider each chakra as a specific language comprehensible to everything in the universe.

Though we may live in a society that does not often recognize us for who and what we are—*spirits attempting to live a human life*—the good news is that neither our spirituality nor the power and happiness we can derive from it depends, of course, on anything or anyone else but ourselves.

Recently I was jogging down one of the mountain roads near my home. I closed my eyes and breathed deeply. I sank my consciousness. I paid particular attention to the chakra behind my heart, for it was this specific energy (or language, or consciousness) that I wanted to share with everything in my environment. I drew chi from all my limbs, favoring that chakra, en route to my center. My chest swelled with high, clean energy, which I sank and extended.

And so what is this thing we call enlightenment?

Of course, it is beyond words. But it is not beyond feeling or knowing. It is our elite experience of being— that which we are all born into, and into which we all have the power to return.

Center yourself. Sit, walk, do anything. Enlightenment is right there with you, wherever you are. Experience it. Listen into the stillness and silence of all things visible and invisible. Call it chi or ki or prana. Call it God. Whatever you call it, get in touch with it. Communicate with it.

You will delight in what you find.

Meditation
Cultivating Spirituality

*The whole universe itself
scattered through the infinities
of space
turns
into enlightenment.*

—DôGEN

The following meditation can be used to heighten your spiritual energies and awareness. You can do it still or moving—that is, seated, walking or running, gardening, or what have you. You choose.

Begin by relaxing yourself. Then center and sink your consciousness downward. Breathe in through your nose. Concentrate on the chakra behind your heart—the point that drives relationships, love, healing, and compassion.

Stimulate that chakra with the stream of your in-breath as you continue to sink your consciousness.

Feel your breast fill with energy. Direct this energy nonspecifically—simply outward into your environment—by projecting your consciousness there. Wait to feel a response. Bring that knowledge with you into everyday life.

Alternate version. Try projecting this energy to something specific, physical or spiritual, in your environment. Wait to feel a response. Bring that knowledge with you into your everyday life.

Resolutions
Cultivating Spirituality

✧ Today, I will listen to the voice of my spirit.

✧ Today, I will be sensitive to the peace I have carried with me since birth.

✧ Today, I will be present; my energy counts.

✧ Today, I will bask in the joy and warmth of my shared consciousness with all things visible and invisible and with the Infinite.

✧ Today, I will see divine presence in everything and everyone.

✧ Today, I will live knowing all things are possible.

Conclusion

*The life of a man is a circle
from childhood to childhood,
and so it is in everything
where power moves.*

—BLACK ELK

The celebration I couldn't have predicted happened about a month after I managed to "tag" my instructor. He had been out of town for several weeks, and when he returned, he decided to test me for my black belt. It was a hot, sunny August afternoon, and the testing was long and strenuous. I worked form after form, drill after drill, technique after technique, from the most basic to the most advanced. There wasn't even a break to drink some water, since the testing wouldn't stop until every skill and every concept had been reviewed. There were points when I didn't think I had the strength to make it through. At times, I actually felt like passing out from heat and exhaustion. I remember having to reach farther inside myself than I'd ever had to go to find the energy to finish.

As with many of my experiences in martial arts, I knew this was a conclusion to a long series of events to which I had committed for one reason and grew into needing for another reason entirely.

What had begun as training in self-defense wound up becoming a journey into my deepest self and a previously unimaginable state of well-being and spirituality. What began as fighting drills wound up training me to experience physical, emotional, and spiritual rapture.

When my testing was over, my teacher asked me to close my eyes and visualize our longest and most beautiful kata. It was one I had practiced thousands of times and from which I'd enjoyed much energy over the years. As I swirled through the movements in my mind, my teacher asked me to hold out my hands. He paused for a moment, then placed my black belt across them. He asked me to open my eyes. And there it was. The belt felt magical in my hands.

My first cycle in the martial arts was complete. I had been changed—reincarnated into a quality of awareness that would nurture me through the rest of my life.

But with every beginning or birth, there is end, and with every end, there is rebirth. Harmonizing one with the other, one moment to the next, keeps us flowing. So, as well as learning how to live, the martial artist must learn how to die all the deaths that life offers in its constant opportunity to change and grow. "The round of summer and winter becomes a blessing the moment we give up the fantasy of eternal spring . . . pleasure is the flower that fades, remembrance is the lasting perfume. . . . To know and to be as though not knowing, that is the height of wisdom," said Bruce Lee. Beginning and end exist side by side. Right next to black is white. This is the continuous cycle of yin-yang. What lingers between them is the perfume of our existence.

The day I earned my black belt was, of course, part of a mutual celebration—mine *and* my teacher's. It marked his own passage toward new experiences as well. He had emptied his cup of knowledge and, as a result, mine had filled. His job was to fill his cup again with new experiences and knowledge. Mine was to share my cup until it emptied.

He told me that I had been his best student, and to symbolize this he wanted to do something special. Thus, he had chosen to pass on to me the same black belt that he had been awarded many years before.

I was honored and humbled.

He then told me a story that beautifully captures the cycle of growth and change—from purity, to experience, and then back to purity.

Traditionally, there were no black belts. All the ancient martial arts masters wore white belts. After years of experience and wear, however, the thick fabric of the white belt soiled and tattered until its

first layer of white eventually turned black. The "black belt" came to be
viewed as a mark of experience, which today we represent with belts
that are dyed black. But like yin-yang, with additional years of expe-
rience and deepened awareness, the ancient masters wore down their
black belts, little by little, to the next layer of fabric, which, of course,
was again white. With that, the cycle was ready to begin again.

Traditionally the contrasting colors of white and black
also indicate the advancement of our spiritual development—which is the ultimate goal of the martial arts.
With this in mind, I ask all of you who have completed
your first passage through this text and adapted its philosophy into your life to close your eyes for a few
moments and rethink your path from beginning to end.
Take your time. Slowly go over all of the lessons that
opened along the way and how each transferred into your
experiences. Remember how each new concept flashed
more light into past ones, further informing your past,
present, and future. This is the way of martial arts. Our
journey lasts a lifetime. The process is synergistic.

When you reopen your eyes, feel the luxuriant energy
emanating from the chakra behind your heart, take a deep
breath, and extend its energy to the world around you.
Tap into that energy often. Speak it to everyone and
everything in the universe.

Our journey has been one of personal growth and

transformation. Your philosophical attainments rank at the level of black belt, to be sure. In this spirit, I wish to celebrate your passage into a new beginning and acknowledge your accomplishments by awarding you your *black belt in life.*

As you continue to grow into these ancient wisdoms, I encourage you to share your knowledge with others; to empty your cup and make room for new knowledge. With each cycle, your skill and spirit will soar to even greater heights. Remember, good energy begets good energy.

Live your black belt in life. Face the world with intensity and enthusiasm. Continue to discover what is. Be present to the goodness of the universe. Live in tranquility and confidence, in touch with yourself and others. Feel comfortable, safe, and free to express your truest self and live your deepest dreams. Be spontaneous and gentle. Live in peace, blissfully and enlightened. Compose beauty in all that you do. Keep flowing.

About the Author

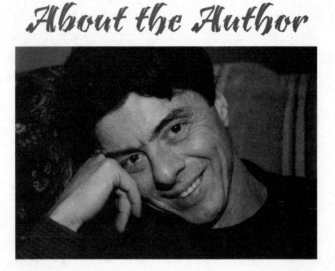

Joseph Cardillo has held the post of head advisor and instructor for the Hudson Valley Community College Martial Arts Club for over a decade. He is a black belt martial arts expert and longtime practitioner of several martial arts including Kenpo Karate, Wing Chun Kung Fu, Tai Chi Chuan, Kali, and Dumog. As a writer, he has taught creative writing for twenty-three years at several colleges, including the University at Albany, where he served as visiting professor in the School of Educational Theory and Practice. At present, he is a full professor of English and Creative Writing at Hudson Valley Community College of the State University of New York. He travels around the country regularly, giving seminars and workshops based on his writings.